Contents

Figures

Tables

Introduction

Public awareness and interest in <u>physical fitness</u> and health is much more obvious today than ten years ago. With today's sedentary and automated lifestyles, nobody can take good health and physical fitness for granted. The way to ensure a lifetime of physical well-being is regular participation in exercise together with a proper diet, adequate rest, relaxation and good health practices.

When good health and fitness have been achieved, the chances are you will feel, look and perform better in leisure and work activities. Perhaps the greatest benefit of being healthy and fit is the degree of independence it affords. Research findings indicate that a fit individual uses less energy than an obese or weak one for any given movement or task. This is most certainly an asset to be prized in one's later years when energy levels may be lower. There is a tremendous psychological advantage in knowing that you can plan and participate in activities without being a liability to colleagues and friends. It is this form of personal freedom that warrants the effort to get and stay fit and healthy.

It was not long ago that regular exercise was virtually the exclusive province of young people. Today, doctors generally recommend it enthusiastically for men and women, young and old alike.

The level of health you can achieve is determined largely by heredity and other factors over which you have little or no control. These include accidents, certain diseases or conditions, and ageing. The extent to which you develop your health potential depends upon your lifestyle. It is most certainly worth the effort to make changes in your living patterns in order to develop positive health qualities. With good health you will be able to live more effectively within your capabilities. Now is the time to start improving your lifestyle.

Health related fitness requires desirable levels of cardiovascular fitness, percentage body fat, flexibility and muscular strength and endurance. These help to prevent the incidence and severity of degenerative types of disease and increase work efficiency.

- Cardiovascular fitness is sometimes referred to as endurance or stamina and denotes fitness of the heart and circulatory system.
- Percentage body fat refers to the proportion of an individual's body weight which is made up from fat. Having too much fat makes the circulatory system work harder and places enormous stress on all body systems.

- Flexibility is the ability to move a joint freely through its complete range of movement. Flexibility can be improved by including stretching exercises daily.
- Muscular strength is the capacity of a muscle to exert force against a resistance.
- Muscular endurance is the ability of a muscle to apply force repeatedly or to sustain a contraction for a long period of time. The longer it can contract without tiring, the better its endurance.

This book is designed to provide information about the beneficial effects of health related fitness. The basic premise is that with proper knowledge and guidance both young and old individuals can design and implement their own positive health lifestyle programmes. They do not have to rely on organised fitness classes. The problem is that when leaving such classes, many people are unable to persist with fitness programmes on their own. This book will help you continue by yourself. It teaches you how to assess, improve and maintain your own fitness. Consideration is given also to health problems such as back pain and bad posture, coronary heart disease, and high blood pressure and stress. Guidance is offered on how to correct or avoid those if you are a sufferer.

This book aims to help you approach health related fitness in a sensible, easy and enjoyable manner.

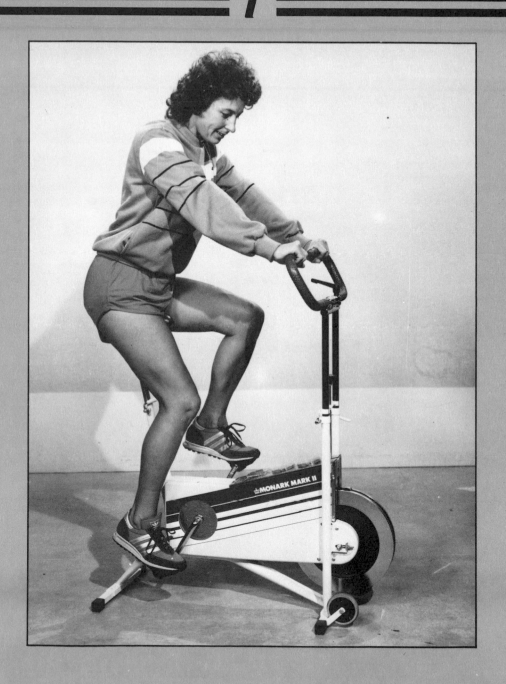

Cardiovascular Fitness

Cardiovascular fitness can be defined as the ability of the circulatory and respiratory systems to supply fuel (in the form of nutrients and oxygen) during sustained physical exercise.

A desirable level of cardiovascular fitness is thought to be the most important component of health related fitness. This is because life depends on the ability of the heart, blood vessels and lungs to deliver nutrients and oxygen to the tissues and to remove wastes via the blood. As a result, exercise has three basic objectives: to enable the lungs to process more air with less effort; to strengthen the heart so that it can pump more blood with fewer strokes; and to increase the elasticity, resilience and internal diameter of the blood vessels so they can manage the greater workload more efficiently.

There is less danger of infiltration of the heart muscles by fat, and of the arteries by cholesterol if the body is kept active. Exercise therefore keeps the efficiency of the heart and the blood vessels to a maximum.

Considerable evidence points to the fact that people who exercise regularly have a lower incidence of heart disease than people who do not. Exercise is also an effective prescription for those who have already suffered a heart attack.

Frequency, intensity and duration

Research has shown that three factors must be considered when designing an exercise programme for developing health related cardiovascular fitness. These three factors are the *frequency*, *intensity* and *duration* of exercise. See Table 1.

Table 1 Frequency, intensity and duration of exercise

Frequency – the number of training sessions per week, per month, per year
Intensity – the training loads per week, per month, per year
Duration – the amount of training in time per week, per month, per year

Fitness improvement is in direct proportion to the *frequency* of training. Programmes on six days per week result in greater improvements than, say, programmes on two days per week. However, to get beneficial results, the intensity, duration and frequency of exercise must be adjusted and suited to each individual.

Warm-up

It is extremely important that you spend ten or fifteen minutes warming up before any training programme. This reduces the risk of muscular injury and pain.

To get the best results, warm-up with movement related to the activity or sport in which you wish to participate. For example, if you are going to perform sprint training, perform the running action slowly and then increase the speed. Flexibility exercises (which will be explained in detail in section three) are recommended too. These will prepare you for the more demanding activity or sport that will take place later on, such as the cardiovascular fitness tests.

Dangers of over-exertion

Never perform physical exercise to the point of complete fatigue or exhaustion. It is dangerous to do this and some of the danger signals are as follows:

a pain in the chest

b severe breathlessness

c dizziness

d light-headedness

e vomiting.

The above symptoms are the body's way of saying that you should stop exercising immediately. If the symptoms do occur then medical advice should be sought.

Regularity of exercise

Regularity of training is very important when engaging in a fitness programme. Top sports' authorities recommend that an individual should receive training stimuli on at least three to five days a week in order to gain and maintain cardiovascular fitness. Regular exercise is the safe way to progress. If you train spasmodically you are courting danger. This type of programme neither develops nor maintains physical fitness. However, a note of warning: if you have a cold or feel poorly you should rest completely. Afer an injury has healed, return to training gently and *not* at the level of intensity you achieved prior to injury.

Footwear

The majority of foot problems are caused by improper shoes or improper use of the foot. Shoes should fit correctly and should never be handed down from person to person.

Two of the most common errors in purchasing shoes are getting them too narrow or too short. Shoes should be at least one centimetre longer than the biggest toe. There should be room also in the widest part of the shoe for the toes and the ball of the foot to spread out comfortably. New shoes should be 'broken in' by wearing them for short periods before extended wear.

The first step in avoiding injury is making the right choice of shoe. Many well established manufacturers provide detailed information which will help you to do this. The second step is not using old shoes. All shoes deteriorate from hard wear and lose their cushioning and support. Excessive wear at the heels is a critical factor. Most runners grind down their heels slightly on the outer side. This gradually tips the foot out of balance. You should repair or replace shoes when they become worn at the heels.

Feet should be washed daily and dried carefully. Socks help prevent friction. They also absorb shock and perspiration. Cotton or wool materials are very absorbent and are good for feet that perspire heavily.

Footwear is an essential investment for the jogger, so make sure what you purchase is comfortable and durable. Look for well-cushioned, well-supported shoes with uppers of a soft, flexible, non-irritating material. Adequate toe room and heel-lift are needed as well.

When to exercise

It is not advisable to train within an hour of eating a meal. Apart from that, almost any time of day is acceptable for physical exercise. It is a good idea to train at the same time each day as this helps establish a regular pattern.

Motivation

Motivation, that something which prompts an individual to act in a certain way, is an abstract factor in learning and performance. It is responsible for:

1 Selection of, and preference for certain activities

2 Persistence in the activity

3 Intensity and vigour of performance

4 Adequacy of performance relative to standards.

To exercise regularly you must be motivated. It is known that performances improve when people understand the value of physical fitness and the physiology of its development and maintenance.

Some people require little encouragement to train while others need constant stimulation. You can get into the right frame of mind by being determined to become physically fit. Be positive. With regular training over a few months, tremendous fitness progress will be achieved. Try to plan your programme intelligently with lots of variety. As people say, variety is the spice of life! Another means to keep you on a regular schedule is to exercise with a friend or your spouse. Meeting a companion and training together helps people to achieve fitness in an enjoyable manner. This provides an added incentive to keep you going.

Cooling down

When you have finished exercising, spend a few minutes cooling down to give your body a chance to recover. This is done best by continuing the activity at an increasingly diminished intensity. For example, if you have been jogging, gradually slow down until you are walking.

Cooling down is important because it allows your muscles to assist in pumping blood from the extremities back to the heart. Since the muscles are no longer contracting and helping to propel the blood back to the central circulation, blood may pool in the muscles. If you stop training abruptly, this could result in insufficient blood to the other organs of the body and cause dizziness to the individual. Therefore, it is sensible to keep moving to help your breathing and heart rate to return to near normal before you head for a well-earned shower or bath. In general, this phase of training should take between 5 to 10 minutes under normal conditions.

The above advice should help to make your exercise programme more beneficial to you.

Cardiovascular fitness evaluations

The tests described and illustrated cover the major areas of cardiovascular fitness evaluation. Although they have limitations, the tests and their results will provide a rough estimate of your state of physical fitness.

1 1½ mile running test One of the best and most accurate measures of an individual's cardiovascular fitness is the maximum amount of oxygen the body can use. This can be measured very accurately in a laboratory, using a treadmill or bicycle ergometer. The gases drawn in from the atmosphere and those expired from the lungs are collected and analysed to determine the body's ability to use oxygen during physical activity.

This procedure is time consuming and not always practical. Fortunately, a simple 1½ miles running test correlates extremely well with laboratory measurements. The time needed to cover the 1½ miles is used to determine the cardiovascular fitness of the individual. Organisation and interpretation of this test is quite simple. In addition, individuals can monitor very quickly their own cardiovascular fitness and that of others. Progress checks can be made periodically by comparing cardiovascular fitness results over time (see *Table 2*).

2 The bench step test

Another simple cardiovascular fitness test is the bench step test. This test must be performed correctly to gain its full benefit.

1 Stand facing a bench (40 cm high for men; 33 cm high for women)
2 Place one foot on bench
3 Step up and place other foot beside the first one. Straighten back and legs so that you are in an upright position
4 Immediately step down again

Continue to step up and down in this manner, keeping time with the cadence of 30 steps to the minute, which is counted aloud as, up, 2, 3, 4, up, 2, 3, 4 and so on. (A metronome will help.) This exercise lasts for 4 minutes or until you can continue no longer. Note how many seconds you have managed out of a maximum of 240.

Now check your pulse rate. The resting pulse rate of adults in general is 72 beats per minute, with children and the elderly faster than this. Men, on average have slower pulse rates than women. Fit individuals have slower rates compared to unfit individuals.

Pulse rates can be found by placing the middle fingers either over the carotid artery alongside the trachea in the

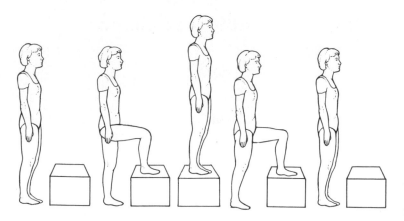

Figure 1 The bench step test   Starting position

neck or over the radial artery on the thumb-side of the wrist. If the carotid artery is used, avoid excessive pressure which may cause the heart rate to slow down by reflex action.

Table 2 Cardiovascular fitness – 1½ mile running test (time given in minutes and seconds)

			Men		
Rating	Age 13–18	Age 19–28	Age 29–35	Age 36–40	Age 41–45
Very good	less than 8:35	less than 9:40	less than 10:00	less than 10:15	less than 10:30
Good	8:35–10:30	9:40–11:45	10:00–12:15	10:15–12:30	10:30–12:45
Average	10:31–12:10	11:46–13:50	12:16–14:40	12:31–15:00	12:46–15:15
Poor	12:11–15:29	13:51–15:59	14:41–16:29	15:01–16:44	15:16–16:59
Very poor	15:30 plus	16:00 plus	16:30 plus	16:45 plus	17:00 plus

			Women		
Rating	Age 13–18	Age 19–28	Age 29–35	Age 36–40	Age 41–45
Very good	less than 11:45	less than 12:15	less than 12:45	less than 13:00	less than 13:30
Good	11:45–13:50	12:15–15:10	12:45–15:40	13:00–15:45	13:30–16:15
Average	13:51–16:45	15:11–17:30	15:41–17:45	15:46–18:30	16:16–19:00
Poor	16:46–18:29	17:31–18:59	17:46–19:29	18:31–19:59	19:01–20:14
Very poor	18:30 plus	19:00 plus	19:30 plus	20:00 plus	20:15 plus

The pulse rate should be counted for a thirty second period exactly one minute after stopping exercise. Note the number of beats. Count again, starting two minutes after stopping exercise and again three minutes after stopping. Make a note. You should have four numbers now. The first is the number of seconds needed for the bench test. The others are the three pulse counts, which should be added together to give a total pulse count. Your score is obtained from this simple formula:

$$\text{Endurance score} = \frac{\text{Duration of exercise in seconds} \times 100}{2 \times \text{the sum of the 3 pulse counts}}$$

For example, if you completed the full four minutes of the test and had pulse counts of 80, 70 and 60, your endurance score would be:

$$\frac{240 \times 100}{2 \times (80+70+60)} = 57.1$$

The endurance score is used as a means of checking your own progress with regular training.

Figure 2 Carotid artery pulse reading

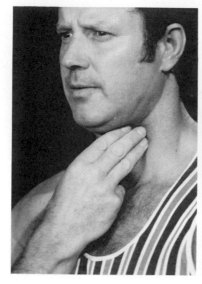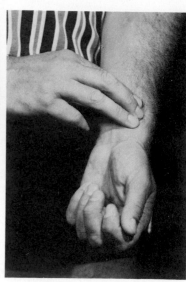

Figure 3 Radial artery pulse reading

Table 3 shows some normal values which have been calculated for young people ranged between 12 and 18 years of age.

3 Bicycle test If the equipment is available, and time permits, then a more scientific test is the bicycle ergometer test.

The test consists of riding a stationary bicycle ergometer for six minutes at a rate of approximately fifty pedal cycles per minute. The workrate will depend on your present fitness and this is usually between 450 to 1,200 kilopond metres per minute (kpm/min) for men and 300 to 900 (kpm/min) for women. It is advisable that a qualified instructor sets the workrate initially.

During the sixth minute of cycling, the rate of heartbeat should be taken. For the test to be valid, the heart rate must have reached the range of 125–170 beats per minute.

When the pulse rate is determined, a nomogram is used to find out the estimated oxygen uptake score. (*See* **Figure 4.**) The point on the right hand scale that represents the

Table 3 Cardiovascular fitness – the bench step test

Endurance score	Rating
90 and over	Excellent
80–89	Good
65–79	Fair
55–64	Poor
54 and below	Very poor

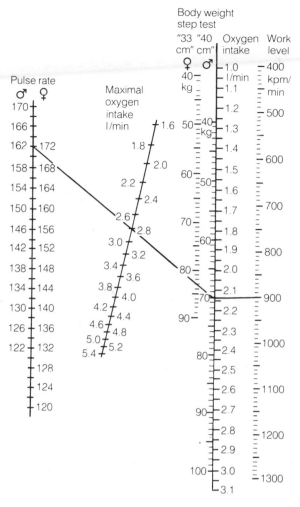

Figure 4 Nomogram – estimated oxygen uptake

Figure 4 shows the nomogram used for estimating maximum oxygen uptake from pulse rate during exercise on the bicycle ergometer[1]. (From Astrand, P. and Rodahl, K. *Textbook of Work Physiology.* McGraw-Hill, 1977 by kind permission.)

Note

In sport science, the kilopond is used as the unit instead of kilogramme force. 1 kp = 1 kgf. One kilogramme force is equal to the force of gravity felt by a mass of one kilogramme on the surface of the Earth.

VO_2 max is a physiological parameter used by sports scientists. It is the maximum volume of oxygen which can be used per minute by the individual.

workrate used in cycling the ergometer is joined horizontally to the oxygen uptake scale. (This indicates the oxygen uptake required for that workrate.) This point is then joined to the pulse rate score on the left hand side of the nomogram. (Do not forget to use the scale marked ♂ for men and the scale marked ♀ for women.) Then look at the estimated VO_2 max reading where a straight line connecting the two points crosses the VO_2 max line (maximum oxygen uptake). Table 4 below shows the cardiovascular fitness classification based on maximal oxygen uptake.

This score provides useful information about the total capacity of the cardiovascular system. Since the value is related closely to body size, we will find that bigger individuals always have much higher scores. To offset this advantage, the maximal oxygen uptake score (VO_2 max) is divided by the weight in kilogrammes (1 kilogramme = 2.2 lb). The resulting score (in millilitres of oxygen per kilogramme of bodyweight per minute) enables us to make a direct comparison of individuals without the problem of different body sizes.

For example, two male participants have the same maximal oxygen uptake score (4.0 litres per minute) but one weighs 80 kilogrammes and the other 100 kilogrammes. The one who has a lower body weight is in a better position to supply oxygen to the muscles and to use that oxygen when it gets there. Therefore, he has a higher level of cardiovascular fitness:

$$4.0 \div 80 \text{ kg} = 50 \text{ ml/kg/min}$$
$$4.0 \div 100 \text{ kg} = 40 \text{ ml/kg/min}$$

This adjustment also gives a more accurate rating for those individuals who are not of average weight.

Even though cardiovascular fitness is one of the most important factors in fitness, 80% of VO_2 max is inherited and cannot be changed. However, with specific training, the VO_2 max can be improved by 15–30% depending on the initial level of training. For example, this can alter a person's rating from poor to above average. This may give an added incentive to participate in such a fitness improvement programme.

Some international sportsmen and sportswomen may have only average VO_2 max scores, yet have bodies which

Table 4 Cardiovascular fitness – the bicycle test (ml/kg/min)

Age (yrs)	Men				Women			
	Very good	Good	Average	Poor	Very good	Good	Average	Poor
20–29	53+	43–52	34–42	Below 30	49+	38–48	31–37	Below 25
30–39	49+	39–48	31–38	Below 25	46+	34–44	28–33	Below 23
40–49	45+	36–44	27–35	Below 22	42+	31–41	24–30	Below 20
50–59	43+	34–42	25–33	Below 20	38+	28–37	21–27	Below 18

compensate for this in terms of superior levels of efficiency and muscular strength and endurance.

To summarise, cardiovascular fitness is one of the most important components of physical fitness. We depend on the capacity of our heart, blood vessels, and lungs to deliver nutrients and oxygen to our tissues and to remove wastes. When the heart and lungs are efficient and functioning effectively, we can perform activities such as jogging, swimming and cycling much better than if we had poor cardiovascular fitness.

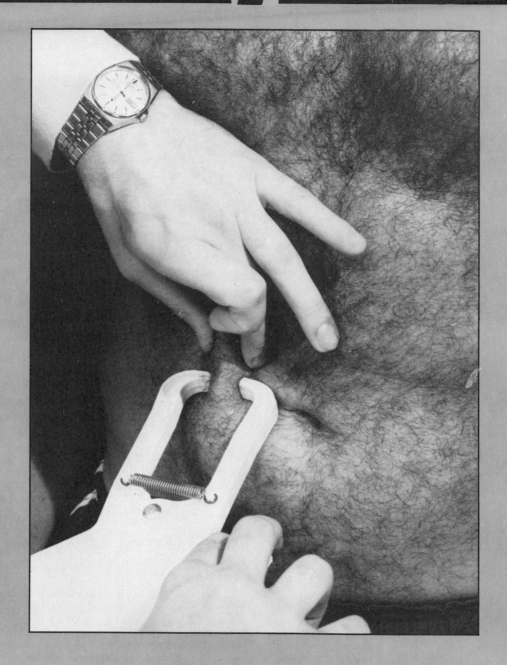

2

Body Composition

There is a saying that 'you are what you eat'. Nutrition does have important implications for your general health and fitness. Proper eating can improve your lifestyle and appearance. It is worth bearing in mind that it is largely you that controls your body shape and size. Nobody forces food down you!

The requirements of good nutrition are relatively simple. They include adequate amounts of energy (calories), protein, fat, carbohydrates and the essential vitamins and minerals.

In a typical normal diet, the carbohydrate, fat and protein should average respectively about 50%, 35% and 15% of daily energy intake. Any food taken in excess can contribute to obesity, which is a health hazard.

Obesity

Obesity is a problem that concerns mainly adults, although it occurs in children as well. Well-filled bodies and moderate stores of fat are advantageous for children and young adults, but definite obesity is a health problem. Being overweight results in disfigurement and inefficiency of physical movement. Moreover, resistance to infectious diseases is lowered and excessive weight places great strain upon the circulatory system and the kidneys. Obese people are more likely to develop functional disorders of the heart, also high blood pressure and diabetes.

Excess fatty tissues may aggravate also types of bone and joint diseases such as osteoarthritis and intervertebral disc problems (back pain). These can cause severe pain. It is therefore important that problems of obesity should be tackled right from childhood. Research suggests that obese children develop into obese adults.

Under-nourishment

On the other hand, undernourishment is particularly serious and a threat to the health of some children and young adults at the stage of rapid growth, i.e. adolescence. Undernourishment may be due to insufficient food, to food lacking in essential nutrients, or to poor utilization of the body processes with the intake of food. Any child who suffers from this kind of symptom is very often highly strung and nervous. Some may be tired and listless most of the time, which is unusual for children and young adults.

Balanced nutrition combined with exercise can help prevent and correct both obesity and undernourishment.

Body type

The factors generally used in evaluating body type (or physique) are the amount of body fat, extent of muscular development and dimensions of body structure. Within certain limits, diet and exercise affect the development of musculature and the amount of fatty tissue but not basic body type. Heredity plays a part in this.

Observation of individual sportsmen and sportswomen shows that body build relates considerably to one's ability to perform. A certain body build may be an advantage or a disadvantage depending upon the nature of the activity or sport. To give an example, height is undoubtedly an advantage in basketball and volleyball. It is less advantageous in gymnastics and weight lifting. A tall and heavy build is an advantage in the shot put, discus throw and hammer throw, but a distinct disadvantage in middle distance running and in many gymnastic activities. Obese people tend to be less athletic although there are some exceptions to this generalization, e.g. Suma wrestlers. People of medium structure with well-developed muscles are generally good performers in such sports as gymnastics, wrestling, weight lifting and swimming. People of slight build tend to do reasonably well in events such as long distance running which require much cardiovascular endurance.

Knowledge that body build and size influence performance in certain ways can be useful to physical education teachers and sports coaches. However, a pupil or sports aspirant should not be deprived of opportunities to excel simply because his or her body build tends to be different from those who usually do well in the sport or physical activity.

Body composition

Body composition can be defined as the relative ratio of fat to fat-free body mass. This composition is assessed and presented as percent body fat.

Assessment of an individual's percent body fat may be through direct body density measurements like water-displacement or underwater weighing methods. However, the easier indirect method uses skinfold measurement. This correlates well with direct measurements.

Nearly one half of all your body fat is situated deep inside your body whilst the remainder is between the skin and the muscles. Body fatness of an individual can be determined quite easily by measuring skinfolds – thickness of fat under the folds of the skin. The instrument used for measuring is called a skinfold caliper.

The skinfold caliper test

All skinfold measurements should be made on the *right* hand side of the body. The skinfold is picked up between the thumb and index finger of the left hand while holding the caliper with the right hand to get a measurement. The caliper should be used about one centimetre from the fingers holding the skinfold and at a depth about equal to the thickness of the fold. Hold the caliper on the skinfold for about three seconds and then make a reading. Measurements are made in millimetres and are read to the nearest half millimetre.

Three measurements should be taken and the average used to determine the final skinfold score. For example, if you had measurements of 10, 12 and 11 your final score would be 11. Here are the skinfold measurement sites:

1 *Triceps*   The measurement is made at the back of the upper-arm, midway between the shoulder and elbow joints. Remember that the arm must be relaxed at all times at the side of the body.

2 *Subscapula*   The measurement is made at the bottom point of the shoulder-blade (the scapula).

3 *Supra-iliac*   The measurement is made just above the top of hip-bone (crest of the illium) at the middle side of the body.

4 *Thigh*   The measurement is made at the middle front side of the thigh, midway between the hip and knee joints. Make sure that the body weight is on the left leg, so that the thigh muscle is properly relaxed.

5 *Abdomen*   The measurement is made at a point adjacent to the umbilicus. (Use a vertical skinfold.)

6 *Chest*   The measurement is made at a point over the outside edge of the pectoralis major muscle near the armpit. (Use a diagonal skinfold between the shoulder and the opposite hip.)

Nomograms predicting body fat

The percentage of body fat can be determined fairly quickly by the use of nomograms such as those illustrated right. These predict body fat for boys (**Figure 11**) and girls (**Figure 12**). Use the triceps and subscapula skinfold measurements to determine the percentage fat for this age group. Although this skinfold test is not perfect, it does provide an estimate of body fatness and is more reliable than the other two sites i.e. thigh and supra-iliac.

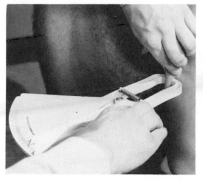

Figure 5 Tricep skinfold

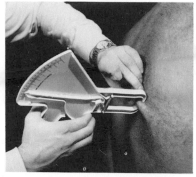

Figure 6 Subscapula skinfold

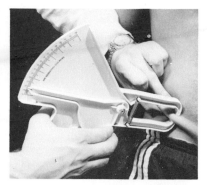

Figure 7 Supra-iliac skinfold

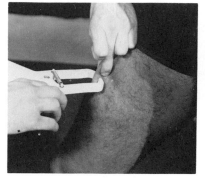

Figure 8 Thigh skinfold

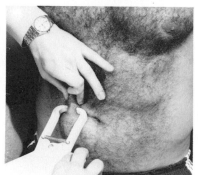

Figure 9 Abdominal skinfold

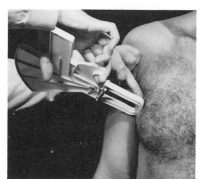

Figure 10 Chest skinfold

Figure 11 Nomogram –
percentage body fat (boys
13–16 years)

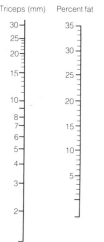

Figure 12 Nomogram –
percentage body fat (girls
13–16 years)

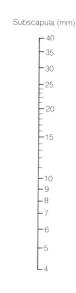

The nomograms for estimation of percentage body fat in children are adapted with permission from 'Total Body Fat and Skinfold Thickness in Children' by Jana Pařízková, from *Metabolism – Clinical and Experimental*, Vol. 106, 1961, pp. 802–805.

For body fat percent prediction, use the nomogram on p. 17. Draw a straight line from the triceps value to the subscapula value. The percent fat is obtained where the straight line crosses the middle column (% fat). For example, a fifteen year old boy with a triceps skinfold of 3 and a subscapular skinfold of 4 would have a predicted body fatness of 5%. Now check this rating with table 5. He is very lean.

Nomograms – Predicting body fat for adults (15–60 years)

To determine the percent fat for adult men 15–60 years, use the sum of three sites (chest, abdomen, and thigh skinfolds) and draw a straight line from these values to the age category. Where the straight line crosses the male column (% fat), this represents the percent fat.

The same procedure is used for women but the skinfold sites of triceps, thigh and supra-iliac are used. (*See* **Figure 13**.)

Table 5 Body fatness rating scale

Rating	Men – percentage body fatness	Women – percentage body fatness
Obese	20 plus	29 plus
Fat	18–19	24–28
Average	14–17	20–23
Lean	11–13	16–19
Very Lean	10 and below	15 and below

Controlling fatness

There are three ways in which an individual can lose weight. These are either by dieting, by exercising or by doing both at the same time.

1 Diet   No single diet plan will work for everyone. Each person must find the diet plan that best suits his or her individual needs. For your own well-being, it is advisable to consult your doctor, or nutritionist first. He or she will analyse your needs and then prescribe a good diet plan for you. However, if you decide to look elsewhere for a diet plan, you should know what to look for. Make sure that the plan you choose takes into account your body's nutritional needs. Diets involving complete starvation or miracle weight-reducing plans do not do this. More importantly, they do not encourage proper eating habits. Individuals on

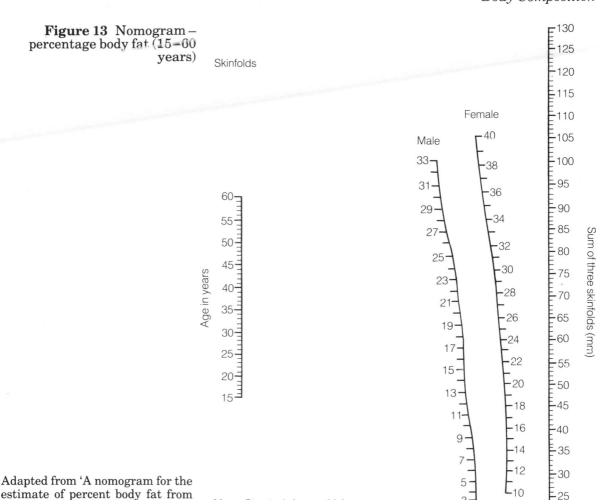

Figure 13 Nomogram – percentage body fat (15–60 years)

Adapted from 'A nomogram for the estimate of percent body fat from generalized equations' by W. B. Baun, M. R. Baun, and P. E. Raven, *Research Quarterly for Exercise and Sport*, vol. 52, 1981, pp. 380–384.

Men : Chest, abdomen, thigh

Women: Triceps, thigh, supra-iliac

these kinds of diets commonly lose a lot of weight at first but then gain much weight back within a few weeks of ending the diet. A good weight-reducing plan offers sound information not only on losing weight but also on maintaining varied meals that will keep you healthy and active.

Proper nutrition guide   It is important to know which foods supply which basic nutrients and how these nutrients are beneficial. The foundation of good physical fitness is a balanced nutritional diet.

Nutrients are the basic chemical elements in food that promote growth, provide energy and are essential to the replacement of worn out cells and tissues. The nutrients are split into five main groups: proteins, carbohydrates, fats, vitamins and minerals.

Proteins are needed for growth, maintenance and repair of body tissues, including bones, muscles and skin. Proteins contain amino acids. These are organic substances that help the body change protein into energy. Foods containing high levels of protein include meat, fish, whole grains, dairy products and some vegetables.

Carbohydrates are a very important and economic source of energy. However, if an individual's diet contains more carbohydrates than are needed, unwanted fat will be deposited within the body. Foods such as rice, cereals, bread, sugar and potatoes contain a lot of carbohydrates.

Fats are another source of body energy. They also help the body to digest food. The body gets necessary fats in two ways. Some fats, such as butter and oil, are added to food. Other fats are already present in food. These include the fats in milk, eggs, fish, meat and nuts.

Vitamins are required only in small amounts although they are essential for growth, maintenance and the repair of body structures. Vitamins are needed as well for regulation of body functions. There are a number of different vitamins and each has a specific function. If one vitamin is missing from your diet, this can cause health problems. The body's vitamin requirements are supplied by a balanced diet.

Minerals are elements in food that promote growth and repair, and regulate body functions. Calcium, iron, phosphorous and iodine are among the minerals that our bodies require.

There are a large number of people who worry about whether or not they are getting enough of these nutrients in their diets. If they are eating balanced meals of basic foods, they should be receiving all the important nutrients required for good general health and fitness.

Major food groups in a balanced diet

To provide a guide for easy diet planning, nutritionists have grouped food into basic categories. These are known as the 'Basic Four' food groups. They are arranged largely according to the nutrients they possess. By choosing items from each group and including them in your daily diet, you can create meals that are balanced, nutritious, attractive and tasty.

Meat and high protein foods

When we eat meat, we are eating the flesh and body tissue of a variety of animals. Cows, pigs, lambs and poultry provide us with the meats most common to our diets. Other common high-protein foods are seafoods, including fish, shrimp, lobster, clams and oysters. We also eat game such as duck, rabbit, deer and pheasant. Other foods included as high in protein are eggs, dried peas and beans, and nuts. Nutritionists strongly advocate one or two servings from this group every day.

Cereals and grain foods   This group includes all the foods made from grains such as wheat, oats, rye, rice, and maize. Grain foods are rich in carbohydrates. Nutritionists recommend four servings from this group daily.

It is not wise to rely on only one or two kinds of food eaten in large amounts. Too much of even a good thing can cease to be beneficial. Only a balanced diet can promote health and such a diet should contain the right variety of foods.

Milk and milk products   This group includes milk, cream, butter, margarine, cheese, cottage cheese and ice cream. Although dairy products supply protein and other nutrients, dairy foods can be detrimental to health if taken in excess. Foods such as butter are rich in saturated fat. Nutritionists advise us to cut down on the total amount of fats we eat, especially saturated animal fats.

Fruit and vegetables   This food group includes all fruits and vegetables. As well as providing essential vitamins and minerals, fruits and vegetables also provide fibre and bulk. This helps the body to eliminate waste normally. We eat parts of plants such as seeds, leaves, nuts, stems and stalks for fibre and bulk. In addition, the outer skins of fruits and vegetables provide fibre and bulk. Nutritionists recommend one or more servings from this group daily.

2 Exercise   A diet that has a variety of foods in sufficient quantity to maintain normal body weight and to support growth is generally adequate for individuals involved in most physical activities. However, there are certain dietary changes needed for people involved in vigorous activities like marathon running.

The quantity of food required by very active men and women varies among individuals from day to day. The establishment of a standard dietary requirement would not be worthwhile. The total daily energy requirement for an active man, for example, may range from 3000 to 8000 calories depending on his size and physical condition and the work performed each day. Exercise expends calories and so can play an important role in controlling body weight.

3 Diet and exercise   If you combine a reduced diet with exercise, the chances of controlling fatness are much better. Note that body weight lost gradually and systematically is more likely to stay off.

Inactivity is the dominant feature in the calorie balance of most fat people. Eating all day without proper exercise leads to overweight. Obesity is not attractive to look at and can lead to health problems. It is vital that individuals are made aware of ways in which body composition can be modified.

Determination of calorie needs

The number of calories needed to maintain proper weight is an individual matter and depends upon a number of factors. These are as follows:

1 Size of the person.

2 Basal metabolic rate. This is higher in men than women and varies with age.

3 Age. Activity and metabolism decrease with age, so about 5% fewer calories are needed each 10 years after age 25 (the average age when growth ceases).

4 Activity. The number of calories used depends upon how many muscles are used and how the activity is conducted e.g. fast, hard and long.

5 Climate – more calories are burned in colder weather than in hot.

6 Pregnancy.

7 Lactation.

8 Temperament – relaxed individuals use fewer calories.

A quick estimation of a person's calorie requirements can be based on the fact that the average person needs approximately 15 calories per pound of body weight. You can arrive at your approximate needs by multiplying your optimum weight by 15. Bear in mind the above eight factors and remember it is only an estimate. The only satisfactory method of determining your need is to ascertain whether you are maintaining your proper weight on that amount. If so, then that is the number of calories you need. If for any reason your weight increases then either your activity or both your activity and calorie intake should be adjusted.

Exercise programmes

There are many different exercise programmes available to help with body weight loss. Any daily paper contains numerous advertisements for weight reduction programmes sponsored by various commercial physical fitness firms. Weight training with sophisticated equipment, slimnastics exercises, aerobic dancing and special exercise apparatus are a few of the approaches often advertised as the best means to lose fat quickly. Remember, to lose body fat the exercise programme should involve large muscle groups, be enjoyable and continuous.

The programme should be designed also to achieve exercise intensity, frequency and duration.

The role of exercise in weight control

The combination of overeating and inactivity leads to increasing levels of overweight. It is generally recognised that prevention of obesity is more effective than treatment. People normally do not become overweight overnight but rather accumulate an extra 75–150 calories per day. That leads eventually to excess fat. An exercise programme carried out regularly can easily offset these unwanted calories.

As the individual's cardiovascular fitness level is increased through training, the amount of work that can be accomplished at a given submaximal heart rate increases. Therefore, the more fit individual expends calories at a faster rate than the less fit individual at a given exercise heart rate.

Basic principles of weight control

People who are interested in body weight control are really interested in body *fat* control. Body fat is nature's way of storing energy in the human body for later use. Body fat control is therefore energy control. To maintain your existing body weight you need to be in energy balance. That is, you must expend as much energy through your daily activities as you consume in your daily diet. Energy output must equal energy input.

During the growth and development period of adolescence, energy input predominates slightly overall causing a positive energy balance and growth of body mass. As adulthood approaches, the major growth processes are virtually complete and energy input and output must be the same. A person will lose weight if the output predominates. This is known as negative energy balance. On the other hand, if the input is greater, a positive energy balance will result and the individual will gain weight. The basic principle to all weight control programmes is proper energy balance.

Figure 14 Energy balance

Too much food input or too little exercise output can result in a positive energy balance or gain in weight. Decreased food intake or increased exercise can result in a negative calorie balance or loss in weight.

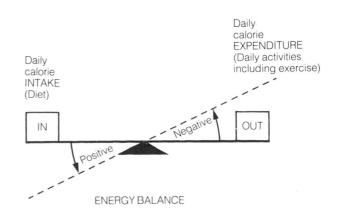

Daily calorie INTAKE (Diet)

Daily calorie EXPENDITURE (Daily activities including exercise)

IN

OUT

Positive

Negative

ENERGY BALANCE

Desired weight How fat you are is more important than how much you weigh in determining your ideal weight. The normal age-height-weight tables are obtained from measurements of many people. These tables help each individual to compare their own figure with that of the average man or woman. These are often an inadequate measure of average weight because of individual variation. For example, many athletes who have little body fat are muscular. They would be overweight according to these tables. In addition, many of these age-height-weight tables allow small increments in body weight with increasing age. This is a practice that lacks justification.

It is the proportion of fat tissue in your body that determines your ideal weight. Skinfold calipers provide a method for measuring the relative leanness or fatness of the body. If these calipers are not available, an alternative is to look at yourself in a mirror and observe if you are fat. If you can pinch about 2.5 cm of flabby fat between your fingers in your midsection, hip region, buttocks and thighs then this is a good indication that you are overweight.

Once you have an estimate of your percentage of body fat (by the skinfold method) you can estimate your desired weight. Body fat values of 18% for women and 12% for men appear to represent reasonable targets for young adults. *(See Table 5 Body fatness rating scale.)*

Figure 15 Facts about weight gain and loss

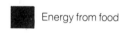 Energy from food

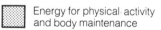 Energy for physical activity and body maintenance

Daily calorie intake   Daily calorie expenditure

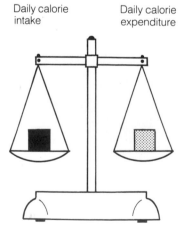

a. Body weight: Stable

(through normal body maintenance with moderate daily activity)

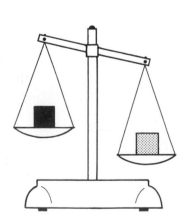

b. Body weight: Loss

(through dieting, vigorous exercise programme, diet and exercise)

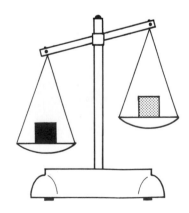

c. Body weight: Gain

(through over-eating, sedentary lifestyle)

Table 6 Calories expended per hour

Activity	Body weight	Calories expended per hour				
		less than 45 kg	less than 57 kg	less than 68 kg	less than 80 kg	less than 91 kg
Archery		180	204	240	276	300
Badminton		255	289	340	391	425
Cycling (normal speed)		157	178	210	242	263
Dance (aerobics)		315	357	420	483	525
Golf		187	212	250	288	313
Gymnastics		232	263	310	357	388
Hiking		225	255	300	345	375
Jogging		485	550	650	750	835
Judo		232	263	310	358	390
Skipping		525	595	700	805	890
Soccer		405	459	540	621	675
Snooker		100	110	130	150	163
Swimming (slow)		240	272	320	368	400
Swimming (fast)		420	530	630	768	846
Table tennis		180	204	240	276	300
Tennis		315	357	420	483	525
Volleyball		204	258	318	372	426
Weight training		352	399	470	541	558
Housework		162	185	243	292	324
Pick and shovel work		268	323	402	482	536
Watching TV		47	56	70	85	94
Gardening		142	170	213	255	284

Calorie expenditure Many activities and sports can help in 'burning up' the calories. Regular exercise is certainly a positive approach to weight control. In addition, as excess weight is removed health risks such as high blood pressure are reduced. For good health and a more enjoyable life, it is strongly advised to stay fit and lean.

Table 6 shows the approximate calorie expenditure per hour for selected activities. If one reads the table, it can be seen that the most calories are expended in activities such as jogging, skipping, swimming, dance (aerobics) and weight training. The least calories are lost through activities involving no exercise at all, such as watching television.

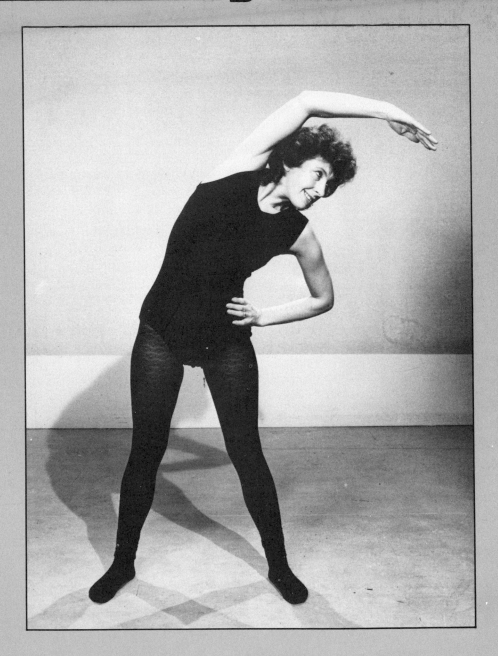

3

Flexibility

Flexibility is an essential component of physical fitness and good performance in sports. Flexibility means an adequate range of movement in all the articulations of the body.

Individuals who have good flexibility can move easily and general movement is not limited. Poor flexibility often hinders movement because of body stiffness.

Limited joint flexibility often contributes to postural problems and increases the risks of developing low back problems. Flexibility is related to age, sex and physical activity. Flexibility decreases progressively with age due to changes in the elasticity of the soft tissue and a decrease in the level of physical activity. It is imperative that older adults should be encouraged to participate in regular flexibility programmes to help offset the loss of elasticity.

How to increase flexibility

Inactivity causes muscles and connective tissue to lose their normal extensibility, thus reducing flexibility. Inactivity may also contribute to body fat accumulation which further restricts flexibility.

Flexibility can be increased by regularly stretching the muscles and the connective tissues.

Two different types of exercises exist to stretch muscles and connective tissues. There is *ballistic* exercise (bobbing) and *slow-tension* exercise (static stretching). Flexibility can be increased by either method. The latter appears to be the more favourable method for the following reasons:

1 There is less danger of exceeding the limits of extensibility of the tissues, which would cause injury and soreness;
2 This method does not activate the stretch reflex; and
3 It provides the opportunity to relax the antagonistic muscles consciously and allow them to stretch.

Exercises that are slow-tension can be performed either passively (with muscles consciously relaxed while another person moves the body segment) or actively (with movement caused by muscle contraction). Passive exercises are extremely beneficial in rehabilitation work but are less desirable than active exercises in sports conditioning.

You should make a particular movement until the stretch pain in the muscles is felt. This position should be held for a few seconds with the muscles consciously relaxed. Favourable results occur when the individual repeats the exercise five to six times daily.

Warm-up first and remember that a stretching exercise should not be performed competitively. If you try too hard, injury can result and with it a loss of flexibility.

Factors which influence flexibility

There are a number of factors which influence your flexibility and the rate at which it can be developed. These factors include activity level, age and sex, body type, specificity of flexibility, stretch reflex and temperature.

Principles relating to flexibility

There are three principles to be observed when considering a scheme of work for flexibility.

1 Overload To increase your flexibility, you must endeavour to stretch muscles further than they are normally stretched. This should be done slowly.

2 Progression To improve flexibility, you must progressively make the exercise harder. Gradually stretch further and perform these exercises for longer each week.

3 Specificity To develop flexibility around a joint, you must exercise that joint. The muscles around it need stretching.

Selection of flexibility exercises

The suggestions that follow represent a selection of exercises that can be incorporated into your fitness programme. These exercises will help you to loosen, stretch and strengthen the main muscle groups of the body.

Arms and shoulders

1 Arm circles Stand upright, with feet slightly apart, arms forward at shoulder level. Lift the arms upwards brushing the ears, and continue circling backwards until the arms have returned to the starting position. Keep the arms straight throughout this movement.

This exercise increases the range of movement in the shoulder region and will help in activities such as swimming (back stroke).

2 Shoulder stretches Stand upright, with feet slightly apart, arms parallel with the ground and folded as shown in **Figure 17**. Move the elbows back as far as they will go comfortably. Count three and then bring the elbows back to the starting position. At all times keep the body upright.

This exercise increases the range of movement in the shoulders. The flexibility will be beneficial in activities that require throwing actions, such as the discus event.

Figure 16 Arm circles

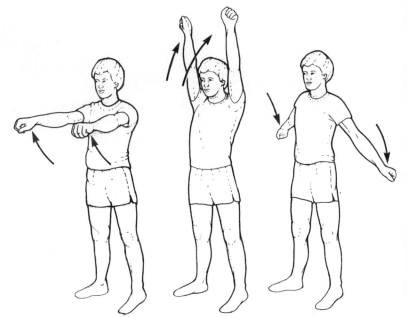

Starting repetitions: 6

Figure 17 Shoulder stretches

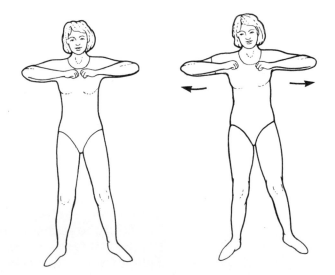

Starting repetitions: 8

Trunk

3 Side bends   Stand upright, with feet slightly apart and hands by the sides of the body. Bend your trunk to the left side and simultaneously slide hand down the thigh and calf as far as possible, keeping the body vertical. Return to starting position and repeat movement on the other side.

This exercise will help to loosen and stretch the side muscles of the trunk. It will help also in keeping the waist trim.

Figure 18 Side bends

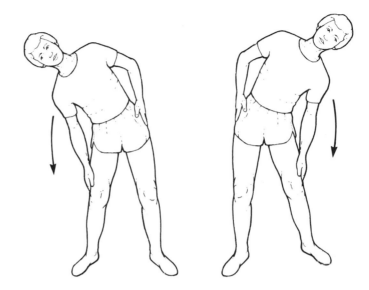

Starting repetitions: 5 each side

4 Trunk twisting Stand upright with your legs slightly bent and a shoulder width apart. With your arms held straight out at shoulder level, twist your trunk as far as you can manage to each side. Perform this exercise **slowly** to prevent injury to the lower back.

This exercise will help to loosen and stretch muscles in the back, sides, and shoulder region. It will improve performance in throwing activities.

Figure 19 Trunk twisting

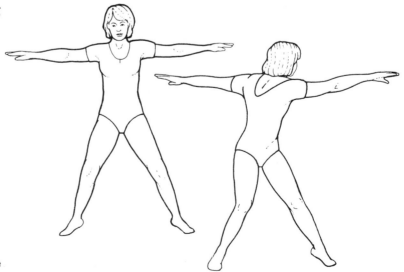

Starting repetitions: 5 each side

Back

5 Low back stretcher Lie flat on the ground. Pull first one knee and then the other to your chest (**Figure 20a**). As a variation on this exercise, you can also hold both knees and bring them to your chest (**Figure 20b**). Hold the chest position for four seconds and then relax. Either keep your head on the floor or bring it forward to your knee.

Figure 20 Low back stretches

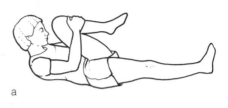

a

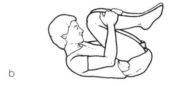

b

Starting repetitions: 5 each leg

This exercise stretches and loosens the lower back and hip flexor muscles. It is often used for rehabilitation purposes for those suffering lower back problems.

6 Arm and leg lift Lie flat on your stomach with your arms stretched away from your head. Raise your right arm and left leg simultaneously and hold them, extended, for three seconds. Return to the starting position. Now raise the left arm and right leg simultaneously and hold these for three seconds. Do this exercise slowly, and repeat at least five times.

This exercise helps to strengthen and stretch the extensor muscles of the back and hip. This is another exercise recommended for rehabilitation purposes.

Figure 21 Arm and leg lift

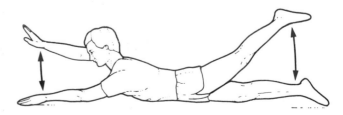

Starting repetitions: 5 each leg

Legs

7 Lunge Stand upright with feet wide apart and hands on hips. Transfer your weight sideways so that most of your weight is on one leg. Hold this position for at least four seconds, feeling a slight stretch on the inner muscles of the thigh. Then transfer the weight onto the other leg for the same time period.

This exercise helps you to stretch the inner sides of the leg muscles and is good for such sports as squash or fencing.

Figure 22 Lunge

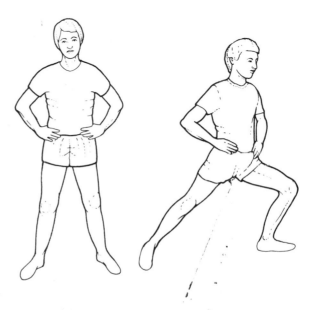

Starting repetitions: 5 each side

8 Inner thigh stretch Sit upright, with legs straight and spread as wide as possible. Bend forward from the hips slowly keeping the top of the thighs relaxed. Keep the hips forward and stretch your hands out in front for support. Press legs into the ground, hold for a few seconds and then relax.

This exercise helps you to stretch muscles in the inner thighs, groin and hip region. It is particularly beneficial for gymnasts, aerobic dancers and athletes.

Figure 23 Inner thigh stretch

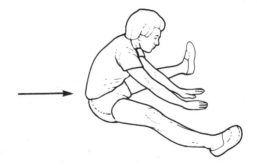

Starting repetitions: 6

9 Calf stretcher Stand facing a wall at arm's distance, legs straight, toes pointing slightly inwards and heels flat on the floor. Lean onto the wall, bending your elbows slowly and keeping your feet flat on the floor. Straighten your arms and return to the starting position. Relax.

This exercise helps to stretch the calf muscles and the achilles tendons. It is especially good as a warm-up exercise before running activities.

Figure 24 Calf stretcher

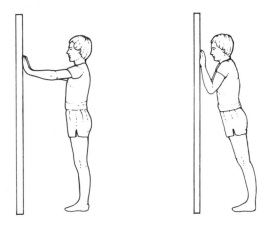

Starting repetitions: 10

10 Side leg raise Lie on your right side, legs extended, with your head resting on your right forearm and hand. Keeping your left leg straight, lift it as high as you can. Return to the starting position and repeat the action at least six times. Change then to the other side and repeat the exercise.

This exercise strengthens and stretches the lateral hip muscles. It is especially beneficial for aerobic dancers.

Figure 25 Side leg raise

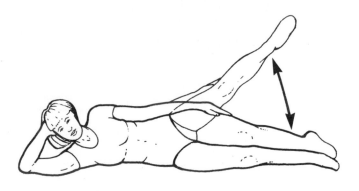

Starting repetitions: 6 each leg

Flexibility test

The sit and reach test for lower back and hamstrings is sometimes considered to be one of the most important single measures of flexibility. It requires little apparatus and is easy to perform. However, if you suffer from back problems then you should not attempt this test.

Sit on the floor with knees together and your feet flat against an immovable object that has a ruler attached to it. (*See* **Figure 26**.) The object of the test is to reach as far as possible down the ruler with the finger tips, keeping the legs straight. The ruler should extend 23 centimetres to the front of the support. Measure the reach to the nearest centimetre.

If you are unable to assemble the measuring device described previously, then the following can be another guide of flexibility in the lower back and hamstrings. Try and touch your toes, bracing the knees backwards. If you can perform this comfortably then your flexibility is adequate. Again, this test is not advisable for people with back problems.

Figure 26 Sit and reach test

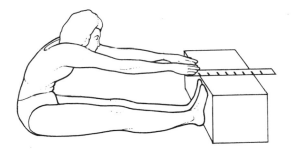

Table 7 Sit and reach test

Rating	Men/Boys cm	Women/girls cm
Excellent	32+	34+
Good	24–31	26–33
Average	17–23	17–25
Poor	9–16	9–16
Very Poor	8 and below	8 and below

Adapted with permission from Corbin, C. and Lindsey, R. *Fitness for Life*, Scott, Foreman and Co, 1983, p. 85.

Guidelines for flexibility

1 Warm up with stretching exercises before your programme.
2 Perform exercises slowly with no jerking movements.
3 Stretch until you feel a slight to moderate discomfort.
4 Hold each stretching position for a brief period.
5 Perform some stretch exercises after your fitness programme to aid recovery.

In summary, flexibility is an important aspect of physical fitness and performance. Flexibility is specific to the person performing the exercise, to the part of the body being exercised and to the type of sport played. The principle of progression should be observed. It is better to begin achieving flexibility gradually than to overdo at first.

Everybody needs a certain amount of flexibility to perform daily chores smoothly. Most young children up to the age of five have extremely flexible joints. It is advisable to try and maintain this flexibility throughout childhood and maturity.

The exercises presented in this section should be performed regularly at a pace and repetition level that suits you personally. If properly performed, they will adequately stretch all major muscle groups and help in muscle and strength development.

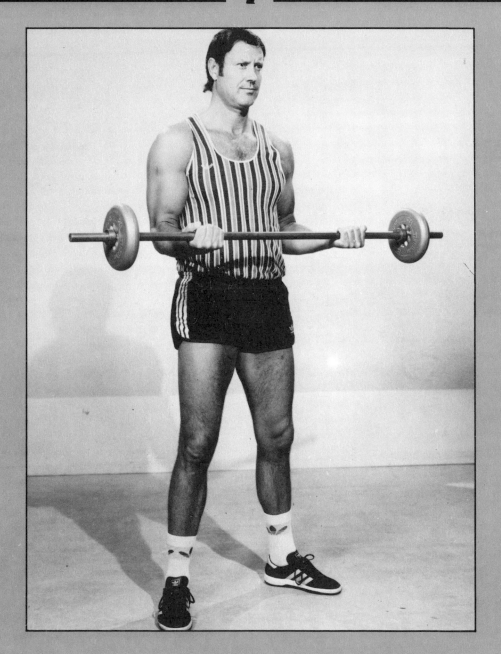

Muscular Strength

Strength is defined as the ability of the body, or particular parts of it, to apply force. It is important to overall body performance in sport and in everyday life. For example, activities such as gardening, shopping, and doing house-work require levels of strength in order to be completed successfully. The general efficiency of the body depends on the condition of the large muscles of the legs, arms and trunk – especially the abdominal and back muscles. If these muscles are weak, then activities will be more difficult. An increase in strength can enhance perform-ance levels for us all.

Strength is built up through resistance. When the movements of muscles are resisted, additional strength is required to overcome the outside forces. The more fre-quently muscles are worked to overcome resistance, the stronger they become.

Resistance – producing equipment (such as dumb-bells, weight machines, barbells, wall pulleys and springs) will improve strength and muscular endurance. There is a misconception that resistance-type exercise develops un-wanted bulging muscles in females. Women's muscles will develop, but since women possess only two-thirds the amount of muscle that men have, they will not develop a masculine physique. Of course, not all men will be able to develop a 'Mr Universe' physique either.

Weight training for strength gains

An effective way to achieve a gain in strength is to follow a programme of progressive resistance exercises. In pro-gressive resistance exercises such as weight training, a muscle is made to contract against a resistance that requires a maximal or near-maximal contraction. Lifting a heavy load a few times generally produces maximum strength and muscle size. Lifting a lighter poundage more frequently tends to produce muscular endurance and good tone. For most people, a programme of the latter is rec-ommended to develop strength and endurance.

Types of strength

There are two types of strength, namely *isometric* (static) and *isotonic* (dynamic). Isometric strength is the ability to apply force in a particular position without going through a range of movement. It involves the static muscle con-tractions involved in pulling against a fixed object like a back and leg lift dynamometer. Isotonic strength is the ability to apply force through the range of movement. It involves dynamic muscle contractions such as the pull-up exercise. Isotonic strength is used more in sport, but the two types of strength are correlated. Isometric strength can be measured more accurately than isotonic strength.

Since strength is so necessary in all activities, it is important to identify where it is lacking and to rectify the condition. Strength tests have been devised for this reason and will be illustrated later on in this section.

Recently *isokinetics* has come to the fore as a type of strength developing programme. Isokinetic exercise combines all the advantages of isometrics and isotonics. It is a programme based on specialized equipment to provide maximal resistance to the muscles (like isometrics) but throughout their full range of movement (like isotonics).

Types of muscle contraction

The term contraction refers to an increase in muscle tension. Muscular contractions are generally classified into different types depending upon whether a muscle shortens, lengthens or remains relatively the same length when contracted. Muscles can engage in three types of contractions, namely *concentric* (shortening), *eccentric* (lengthening) and *static* (no change in muscle length).

Concentric contraction

This occurs when a muscle develops sufficient tension to overcome a resistance, thus causing a visible shortening and movement of a body part. The muscle actively shortens and thickens with the insertion usually approaching the origin. (The origin is that part of a muscle which remains relatively fixed during a movement under normal circumstances. The insertion is that part of the muscle which moves a bone and is usually the distal attachment.)

An example of concentric muscle work occurs when bending the elbows to bring the hands in front to the chest (two arm bicep curl). In this case the resistance of the forearm and the effects of gravity have been overcome by the flexors of the elbow working concentrically. That is, they shorten so that movement takes place.

Eccentric contraction

This type of contraction occurs when the origin and insertion of a muscle are drawn further apart under control, either by the effects of gravity or some other outside force. The muscle actually becomes longer and thinner, but still remains firm because it is working. Such gradual releasing or 'letting-go' occurs either when gently lowering a weight under control or when the outside force is greater than the force of the contracting muscle. Although the term 'lengthening' is generally used to describe this type of muscle contraction, what actually happens is that the muscle returns to its normal resting length from its shortened working position. An example of eccentric muscle work occurs when outstretched arms are slowly lowered from the front to the side of the body.

Static contraction Static contraction occurs when a muscle increases in tension but causes no appreciable joint movement. The length of the muscle remains the same, although either a maximal or sub-maximal contraction may be made. Static contractions can occur also when muscles antagonistic to each other contract with equal strength, balancing or counteracting each other.

An example of static muscle work is holding arms outstretched to the sides, parallel with the ground. Static contractions can be made with gravity eliminated by, for example, lying down and tensing the quadriceps (the muscles on the front of the thighs).

The term *isotonic* (equal tension) is used often to describe concentric contractions. However, an isotonic contraction is one in which the tension remains the same as the muscle shortens. A concentric contraction involves a decrease in muscle length. *Isometric* (equal length) contractions are often associated with static contractions. Isometric contractions are those which occur when a muscle is unable to shorten due to the magnitude of the resistance, as distinct from merely counterbalancing the effects of gravity. Only when static contractions involve maximal efforts are the two terms used synonymously.

Principles of weight training

Some of the principles relating to weight training include overload, progressive resistance, specificity, exercise sequence and recuperation. Improvement in strength will come more quickly, and with less chance of injury, if the exercises are performed in certain ways. A good programme is one which provides the principles mentioned above.

Overload The overload principle is perhaps the most important in all weight training programmes. To become stronger, the muscle must work harder than normal. This is accomplished by selecting resistances heavy enough to cause the muscle to work to a certain capacity, and then progressively increasing the resistances as the muscle becomes stronger.

Progressive resistance In order to get stronger, you must increase the amount of resistance (overload) in your training programme so that you provide the proper stimulus for muscle growth. This is known as progressive resistance. Weight lifting is usually performed in repetitions and sets. A repetition is one complete exercise while a set is a number of repetitions of the same exercise performed continuously. There is no single best combination of sets and repetitions, but usually 2 or 3 sets with 5–10 repetitions provide an adequate stimulus for muscle growth. A recommended combination for beginners is 3 sets with 5 repetitions in each set. The very first thing to do in each individual exercise is to determine the maximum amount of weight that you can lift for 5 repetitions. If you can manage to do more than 5 repetitions, the weight is too light and should be increased. As you get stronger during the following weeks you should be able to lift the original weight more easily. When you can do 10 repetitions, increase the weight so that you go back to 5 repetitions again. This is the principle of progressive resistance. Over a period of time, the weight will need to be increased many times as you continue to become stronger.

Specificity
This principle has many implications for weight training, including specificity for various sports movements, strength gains, endurance gains and body weight gains. In order for a particular muscle or muscle group to increase in size, the weight training programme must be designed specifically to achieve this end. Perhaps the most important aspect of training specificity is to develop a programme designed to meet the needs of a given individual.

Exercise sequence
The weight training programme should be based upon the principle of exercise sequence. For example, if you have 6 exercises in your training programme, they should be arranged in such an order that fatigue does not limit your lifting ability. As an illustration, the first exercise in a sequence of 6 might stress the arms and shoulders, the second the trunk, and the third the legs and so forth. After you complete one set of the 6 exercises, you then perform a second set followed by a third set.

Recuperation
If you perform your weight training exercises properly, then severe stress is imposed on the muscles, requiring a period of recovery or rest. In particular, beginners should generally do weight training on only about 3 days a week (say, Mondays, Wednesdays and Fridays). Following this type of schedule allows your body sufficient time for muscle growth and helps to prevent undue muscular fatigue.

The above general points of weight training should serve as guidelines during the commencement of your weight training programme.

Strength and power

A great deal of confusion exists in popular literature dealing with weight training. Uninformed writers often use the terms strength and power as though they were interchangeable. They have quite distinct meanings. *Strength* refers to the ability to produce or resist a force. *Power* refers to the rate at which such work is done. It is determined from the amount of work done and the time taken to do it. Power = strength (force) × speed (velocity). Power would be greater if a given weight were lifted quickly rather than slowly, although the strength involved would be the same.

Safety considerations

Safety in weight training is more than merely avoiding major accidents. There are many aspects to safe training, including the prevention of sprains, strains, tears and other soft tissue injuries. Safe training procedures concentrate on three general areas, namely equipment, space and technique.

1 Equipment All equipment should be in good working order and checked periodically for wear and tear. Safe equipment implies tight fitting collars which stay in place on the barbells and dumb-bells during exercises, and exercise machines that operate smoothly during use.

Proper adjustment for the person using the equipment, particularly apparatus such as the multi-gym, is also important. These machines are designed carefully to accommodate individual differences. Limb lengths for example, should always be repositioned for each new user. The time taken in making these adjustments is time well spent. It increases the muscle training effects and decreases the possibility of injury.

2 Space Weight training requires much more space than most people imagine. Adequate space is needed for free-weight exercises in which barbells and dumb-bells are moved in every direction. Space is needed also around exercise machines and this should be remembered as well. Moving pulleys, cams, cables and weight stacks can cause serious injuries if someone steps too near or leans against a machine carelessly. In addition, calisthenic types of exercises such as sit-ups, pull-ups, bar dips, and push-ups need sufficient amounts of space if they are to be performed correctly and safely.

The safe weight training area should be spacious and uncluttered. Exercise stations should not be too close together and there must be room to allow easy movement between them. There must be enough space to accommodate people who are lifting, stretching, warming up, cooling down, discussing their training and making notes in their training diaries. Every piece of equipment should have its own particular place for storage and for use. Neatness and orderliness will help ensure safety too.

3 Techniques Many accidents in the weight room occur as a consequence of improper training techniques. In addition, unsupported exercises such as the standing press carry a higher risk of injury than supported exercises such as the bench press. Figure 27(b) illustrates the stress area of the lower back imposed by unsupported overhead pressing movements.

Figure 27 Comparison of overhead pressing movement

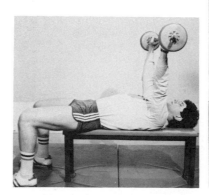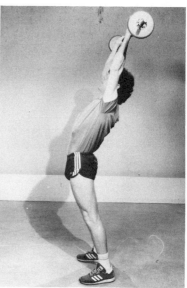

Note the hyper-extension of the lower back in the unsupported standing press.

Most muscle injuries result from a lack of attention to basic biomechanical principles. Unfavourable leverage arrangements are mostly responsible for subjecting the lower back muscles to high stress in exercises.

Poor technique is an inevitable consequence of incorrect positioning on an exercise machine like the multi-gym. It is therefore important to make the appropriate adjustments prior to performing repetitions on a mechanical exercise machine.

Poor technique is exhibited frequently during attempts at personal weightlifting records. Hip lift on a bench press and arching on a standing two arm curl are common movements that permit heavier lifts but place tremendous stress on the lower back. (*See* **Figure 28**.)

Injuries tend to be quite severe due to the intensity of most weight training exercises. Several weeks of rehabilitation are often needed. It is extremely important to be safety-conscious in the weights room. A debilitating injury may prompt many novices to give up weight training altogether. Periodic equipment checks, sufficient training space and correct exercise techniques are the keys to safe and enjoyable weight training programmes.

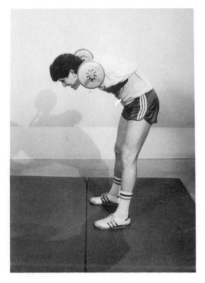
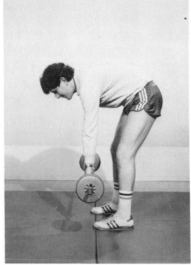
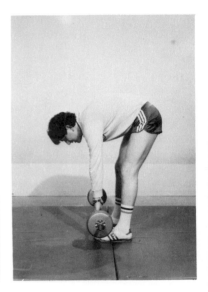

Figure 28 Three exercises that subject the lower back to stress

Stress is due to unfavourable leverage factors

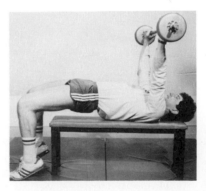
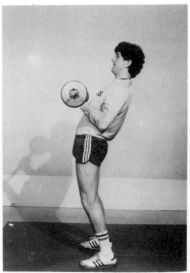

Incorrect technique in these exercises places great stress on the muscles of the lower back.

Figure 29 Incorrect technique – bench press and two arm curl

Additional safety precautions for the individual

1 Weight training is great fun because you can see and take pride in the progress you are making. However, it takes time to become an expert. You must understand and master each step before moving on to the next. Don't try to run before you can walk.

2 Before attempting new exercises or training plans and schedules, seek and follow advice from your teacher or coach.

3 Whenever possible, train with a partner for safety and encouragement.

4 Keep to your schedule of exercises. Do not advance to greater weights without your coach's advice. Do not sacrifice correct technique for extra kilogrammes.

5 Try not to compare yourself with others. Each person develops muscular strength at their own rate (due to inherent physiological and biomechanical factors).

6 Do not fool around in the weight room as it is extremely dangerous.

7 Inhale and exhale with each repetition. Do not hold your breath when lifting weights.

8 Check all apparatus before use and after each exercise. Check collars. Make sure they are firmly secured. Make sure all bars are loaded evenly. Concentrate and be safety conscious.

9 Older people should consult their doctor before they begin to train with weights. Children under fourteen should not do weight training.

10 Lift weights with a straight/flat back at all times.

Strength training equipment

Many health and fitness clubs possess equipment that would please any strength and fitness training enthusiast. The equipment may include isokinetic machines, conventional barbells and dumb-bells (free weights), multi-gyms and strength testing machines. The choices are varied. All that is needed for success in strength development is hard work. Here is just a basic introduction to some strength training equipment. It is beyond the scope of this book to talk about these in more detail.

Barbells and dumb-bells (free weights)

Barbells and dumb-bells have been the basis of strength training programmes for years. They are still the most familiar and widely used types of exercise equipment. They are known also as free weights because they are not attached to fixtures or machines. Free weights can be manipulated by the exerciser in any way desired.

Free weights can be used for both concentric contractions (positive work) and eccentric contractions (negative work). However, due to the fact that the muscles and bones of the body function as lever systems, the same weight may feel lighter in one position than in another. All free weight exercises have a so-called 'sticking point'. This is the point in the range of movement at which the mechanical factors are least favourable and the greatest amount of muscle force is required. It is the point where the exerciser succeeds or fails in making the lift.

As an illustration, the 'sticking point' in the bench press exercise is near the chest, as shown in **Figure 30**. Greater muscular effort is required at this point than at any other due to the mechanical factors involved. As soon as the barbell is pressed beyond the 'sticking point', less muscular effort is needed to complete the lift. The body's lever arrangements then become more favourable for lifting.

Figure 30 Position requiring greatest muscular force for bench press

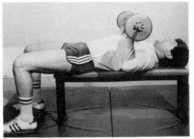

Multi-gym Multi-gyms are designed to provide a wide range of compact exercises for different parts of the body where space is minimal. The variety of exercises includes those which may be done simultaneously by a group of people. Some multi-gym units have eighteen or more exercise stations. There are also many varied single unit exercise stations, some of which may allow several exercises to be done.

The different types of multi-gyms provide facilities for a great number of exercises, dependent to a certain extent on the number of exercise stations they contain. The possible exercises include the bench press, leg press, shoulder press, sit-ups, back extensions, rowing, hip flexion, knee extension and flexion, and tricep dips. These and many other exercises can be done with varying levels of resistance.

Multi-gyms have certain inherent advantages over other conventional training devices. They are a great space saver yet are able to cater for several people at once. They are portable and require little or no fixing. Storage poses no problems. They are safe to use and are found in all sorts of institutions as well as sports centres. Above all, they are fun to use and provide a wide variety of exercises.

A selection of weight training exercises

Weight training exercises can be classified into three categories – namely, power, strength, and general fitness and mobility exercises. Power and strength can be developed from fast, rapid movements while slower movements develop strength and full mobility. The way in which an exercise is executed, and the number of repetitions and sets required, depends on whether power, strength or mobility is wanted. Another point to bear in mind is the choice of exercises in a given programme in relation to both the preceding exercise and the rest interval taken between exercises.

The few basic exercises mentioned in this section are in a specific order. It is hoped that an adequate and varied schedule can be devised to suit individual needs. Keep in mind the weight training objectives and the nature of your own sport or fitness aspirations when compiling a schedule.

Breathing technique

Correct breathing technique plays an important role in executing weight training exercises. It must be practised if maximum effect is to be achieved. However, opinion varies as to the best moment to inhale. Oxygen is necessary for muscular activity. Inhalation needs to have taken place in order to exert maximum effort during the pushing, pulling or lifting phase of an exercise. It would be difficult to hold a strong position (i.e. one with a heavy weight) with deflated lungs. The author believes that inhalation should take place just before the phase of greatest exertion. For example, when pressing a barbell overhead from the chest, inhalation should be immediately prior to raising the barbell. Exhalation should be when the elbows lock or when the barbell is lowered to the chest. It is advisable to breathe during each repetition rather than hold your breath for a given number of repetitions. Many exercises include two stages, one to achieve the starting position and one to execute the exercise itself for a given number of repetitions before returning the barbell to the floor. Correct breathing technique plays an important part in both stages of any exercise. Such technique should be observed with regard to the selected exercises in the next few pages. Most of those exercises using barbells and dumb-bells have counterparts on the multi-gym. The exercises should be performed in the order in which they appear here.

1 *The bench press*
(chest)

This exercise is an extremely popular one amongst weight trainers as it helps to develop the power and strength of the chest and arms. It is also a good conditioner.

Bench press	
Muscles involved	Pectoralis major, deltoid, triceps
Sets	4–5
Repetitions	5–10
Safety	Have two spotters standing at the sides of the bar
Movement	Back-lying. Use wide grip for the development of the chest muscles. Press the bar upwards slowly to full arm extension and then lower slowly to the chest. As a safety precaution, do not arch the back.

Figure 31 Bench press

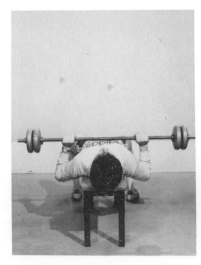 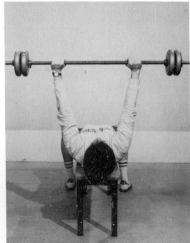

2 Two arm curl (fronts of the upper arm)

This is a popular exercise for men. When **performed** correctly, this exercise emphasizes the role of the biceps muscle and enables the use of relatively heavy resistance. The key to obtaining the best results from this exercise is to keep the upper arms stationary whilst the lower arms go through a full range of movement.

Two arm curl

Muscles	Biceps plus several elbow flexors
Sets	4–5
Repetitions	5–10, using progressive resistance method
Safety	Keep body straight throughout movement
Movement	Stand upright, with feet shoulder-width apart. Bend the elbows. Bring the barbell to the chest and then lower it slowly to the starting position.

Figure 32 Two arm curl

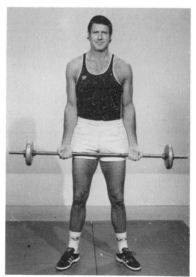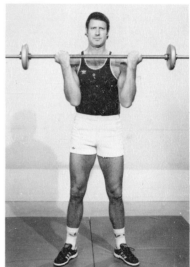

3 The power clean (all round physical development)

The power clean is a powerful and important exercise suited to most sportsmen and sportswomen. It is also an excellent explosive exercise developing body power.

The power clean

Muscles involved	Gastrocnemius, quadriceps, gluteus maximus, erector spinae, biceps and deltoid
Sets	3–4
Repetitions	5–8, using progressive resistance method
Safety	Pull in a straight line – not backwards
Movement	The exercise starts by squatting behind the barbell and taking an overhand, shoulder-width grip on the bar. With the arms extended and the back straight, the performer lifts the barbell off the floor with the legs. The bar is pulled upward in a straight line until the elbows are as high as possible. When the barbell reaches its highest point the elbows are swung forward and the bar is caught in a shoulder rest position. After a slight pause, the barbell is returned to the floor in a controlled way.

Figure 33 Power clean

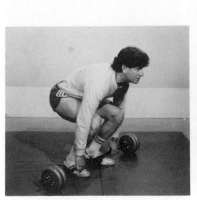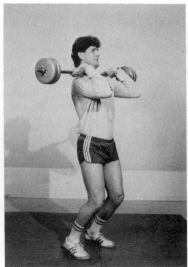

4 The half-squat   This is a classic exercise for the development of the legs.
(legs and thighs)   The exercise can be performed with relatively heavy
weight loads and requires a squat rack and two spotters.

The half-squat

Muscles	Quadriceps, hamstrings and gluteus maximus
Sets	4–5
Repetitions	5–10, using progressive resistance method.
Safety	Have two spotters at the sides of the bar. Do not squat more than half-way down.
Movement	From an upright stance, squat until thighs are parallel with the ground, keeping the back as straight as possible. Return to the standing position.

Figure 34 Half-squat

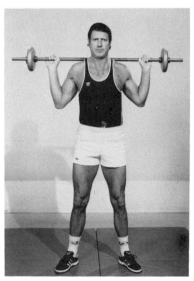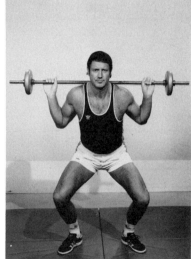

5 *Lateral raise*
  (shoulders)

This is an extremely good exercise for the development of the deltoid muscles of the shoulders.

Lateral raise

Muscles	Deltoid and trapezius
Sets	4–5
Repetitions	5–10, using progressive resistance method
Safety	Keep back straight throughout the movement
Movement	Stand with dumb-bells in hands at the sides of the body and feet slightly apart. With palms down, raise straight arms sideways to shoulder level. Return slowly to the starting position.

Figure 35 Lateral raise

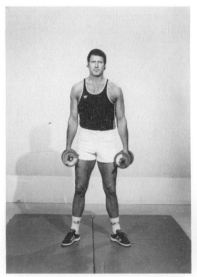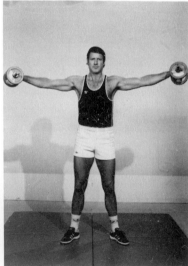

6 Calf raise
(calf muscles)
This exercise develops the calf muscles and is popular with people who include running activities in their sport training programmes.

Calf raise

Muscles	Gastrocnemius and soleus
Sets	4–5
Repetitions	5–10, using progressive resistance method
Safety	Have two spotters at the sides of the bar
Movement	With the bar on the back of the shoulder, rise up on your toes as high as possible, and then return to the starting position. Place toes on a board or two discs so heels can drop down lower than usual.

Figure 36 Calf raise

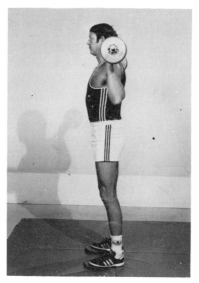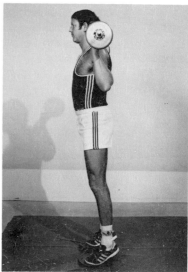

7 Press behind neck (shoulders and back of arms)

This is an excellent exercise that develops shoulder mobility. It is a must for enthusiasts developing their strength.

Press behind neck	
Muscles	Triceps, deltoid and trapezius
Sets	4–5
Repetitions	5–10, using progressive resistance method
Safety	Keep back straight throughout movement
Movement	Stand upright with feet apart, the bar behind the back of the shoulders. The hands should be slightly more than shoulder-width apart. Press the barbell overhead until the elbows lock and then lower the barbell slowly to the starting position.

Figure 37 Press behind neck

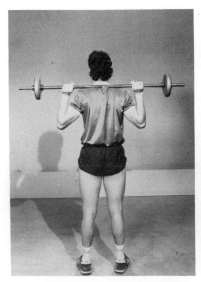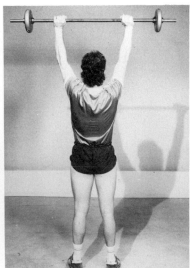

8 *Dumb-bell side bend*
  (abdominals, trunk)

This exercise helps to tone and trim the sides of the trunk.

Dumb-bell side bend

Muscles involved	Obliques, sacrospinalis
Sets	4–5
Repetitions	8–12 either side, using progressive resistance method
Safety	Do not bend towards the feet during the movement
Movement	In an upright position, take hold of the dumb-bell in one hand and place the other hand behind the head with elbow pointing sideways. Bend from the waist and lean to the dumb-bell side as far as possible, keeping the body square at all times. Return to upright position and repeat. After several repetitions change hands to exercise the other side of the body.

Figure 38 Dumb-bell side bend

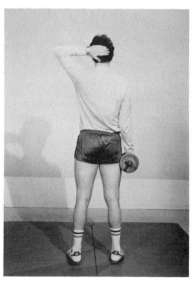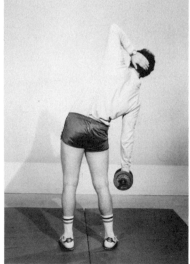

9 Upright rowing (shoulders and fronts of the upper arm)

This is a good exercise for the development of shoulder strength.

Upright rowing	
Muscles	Deltoid, brachialis, biceps.
Sets	4–5
Repetitions	5–10, using progressive resistance method
Safety	Keep body straight throughout movement
Movement	Stand upright and grip (overgrasp) with hands 15–20 cm apart, arms in front of body. Pull the barbell to the chin keeping it close to the body. Keep the elbows above the hands at all times. Lower the barbell to the thighs and repeat movement.

Figure 39 Upright rowing

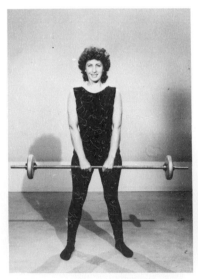 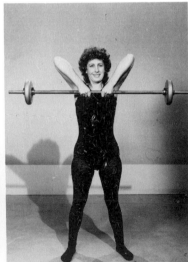

10 *Sit-ups (abdominals)*   This is an excellent exercise for obtaining a flat and hard stomach. The sit-ups strengthen the rectus abdominis as well as the obliques.

Sit-ups	
Muscles	Rectus abdominis, internal and external obliques
Sets	4–5
Repetitions	5–10, using progressive resistance method. (If you do not use weights, then increase the number of repetitions.)
Safety	Develop sufficient abdominal strength before using weights with this exercise. Do not arch back when exercising.
Movement	Lie on your back with knees bent, hands holding weight on the chest. Sit up about half-way and then return slowly to the starting position.

Figure 40 Sit-ups

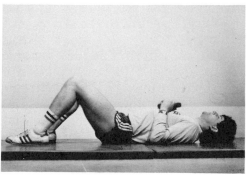 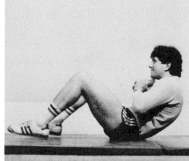

Keeping records A weight training record sheet, similar to the one illustrated in *Table 8*, should be used to keep you and your instructor informed of progress made with each exercise.

Table 8 Weight training record sheet

Name	Body Weight	Activity/Sport

Duration of Training	From:	To:
Date		

Exercise
Sets
Reps
Kg

Instruments for strength measurement (static)

The back lift and leg lift dynamometer and the hand dynamometer are instruments designed specifically to measure strength in these parts of the body.

The back lift and leg lift dynamometer is a dial with a chain and bar attached, mounted on a platform. To use it, you hold the bar, standing on the platform, and apply force upwards. The dial indicates in pounds or kilogrammes the amount of force exerted. This instrument measures the strength of the leg or back muscles, depending on how the force is applied. The hand dynamometer tests right and left hand grip strength.

The following tests are particularly useful as they are easily administered.

Leg lift test This test measures the strength of the leg extensor muscles and is a good indicator of total leg strength.

Hold the bar with both hands, palms down (overgrasp) so that it rests on the front of the upper thigh. Maintain this position while the belt is fastened to the handle and adjusted. Bend knees slightly and alter your stance on the dynamometer platform so that the movement will be directly upward when you pull. The chain length is now adjusted. Then, at a signal from the teacher or instructor, exert a maximum force upwards by extending the legs, keeping the arms and back straight.

Make two attempts, and record the best of the two to the nearest pound or kilogramme.

Figure 41 Leg lift strength test

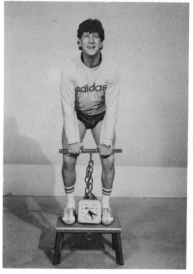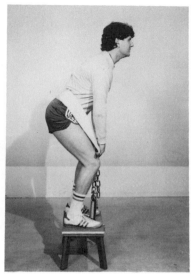

Back lift strength test This test measures the strength of the back extensor muscles.

Stand in position on the dynamometer platform. When the chain length has been adjusted properly, bend forward and grip the bar with one palm facing upwards and one facing downwards. Keep legs straight, feet flat on the platform and head and eyes looking forward. When indicated by the teacher/instructor, lift steadily with maximum force. Scoring is the same as for the leg lift test. (Figure 42 shows a grip variation.)

Figure 42 Back lift-strength test

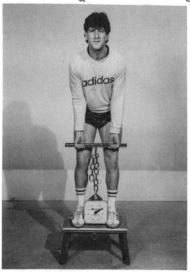

Hand grip strength test This test measures the grip strength of the right and left hands. The only equipment needed is a hand grip dynamometer.

Hold the dynamometer in the palm of the hand with the arm by the side of the body, palm facing inwards. Grip the dynamometer with maximum force and then read the score on the dial of the dynamometer. Perform this test twice with each hand and take the best reading as the final score.

Table 9 *Static strength norms (kilogrammes)*

Rating	Left grip		Right grip		Back strength		Leg strength	
	Men	Women	Men	Women	Men	Women	Men	Women
Very good	>60	>35	>65	>40	>200	>105	>240	>135
Good	50	30	60	35	180	100	210	130
Average	45	25	50	30	160	75	180	100
Poor	40	20	45	25	120	45	150	60
Very poor	<35	<15	<40	<20	< 95	<40	<140	<50

If you are left-handed simply transpose the figures given for left grip and right grip in *Table 9* above.

Figure 43 The hand grip dynamometer

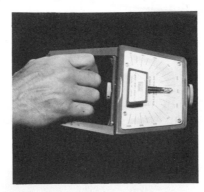

Dynamic strength tests

Pure dynamic strength is difficult to measure. Maximum lifts with weight training equipment generally provide the best results. A lot of experimenting is needed to determine the greatest weight you can lift at once.

Dynamic strength and endurance tests Movements against one's body weight, such as pull-ups, have been used as measures of dynamic strength. However, these tests do not measure pure strength but rather a combination of strength and endurance. There are many muscular strength and endurance tests that are possible in limited space and with little or no special test equipment. Such tests provide an immediate sense of satisfaction as you see yourself achieving better results.

Muscular power test: vertical jump

This is a test of all-round power. It is frequently used by athletes in training to periodically check improvements in the explosive power of their legs.

Face the wall with both feet flat on the floor. Reach as high as possible with either hand and make a chalk mark on the wall or a jump board, if one is available. Now jump as high as possible from any position. At the peak of jumping, make another chalk mark above the first one. Measure the distance between the two to the nearest centimetre. Do the test three times and record the scores.

To determine your vertical jump rating use Table 10.

However if bodyweight and the speed in performing the jump are not a part of the measurement, one cannot regard this test as a true measure of power. For example a 70 kilogrammes boy who jumps vertically 60 centimetres produces less power than the 80 kilogrammes boy who jumps 60 centimetres.

In order to make the vertical jump test more valid as a measure of leg power, the adjusted Lewis nomogram (Figure 45) can be used. Power output can be determined linking the jump reach distance on the left to the performer's weight on the right with a straight-edge. The power output is then read off on the central scale where the line crosses.

Figure 44 Vertical jump test

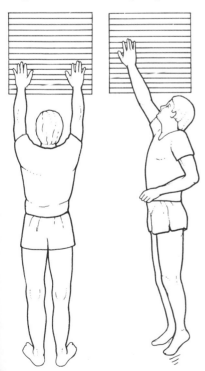

Table 10 Vertical jump rating scale (cm)

Rating	Men			
	Age 15–20	20–30	30–40	40–50
Poor	32	38	36	30
Fair	42	48	45	38
Average	50	54	52	44
Good	55	60	57	50
Excellent	60	65	62	56
Rating	Women			
	Age 15–20	20–30	30–40	40–50
Poor	30	32	25	20
Fair	38	40	32	25
Average	42	44	40	32
Good	50	52	46	40
Excellent	55	57	52	46

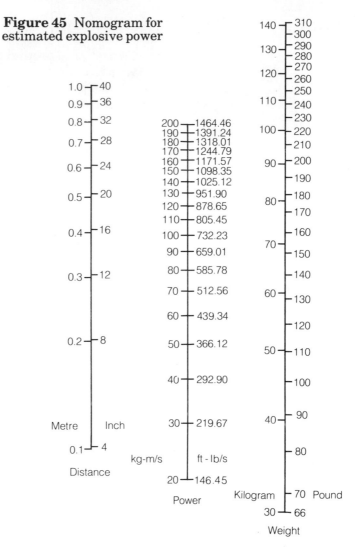

Figure 45 Nomogram for estimated explosive power

To summarise, a sufficient amount of muscular strength is important for everyone. It is needed especially by those following some occupations and leisure pursuits. Reasonably toned and strong muscles make you more effective in whatever you do.

5

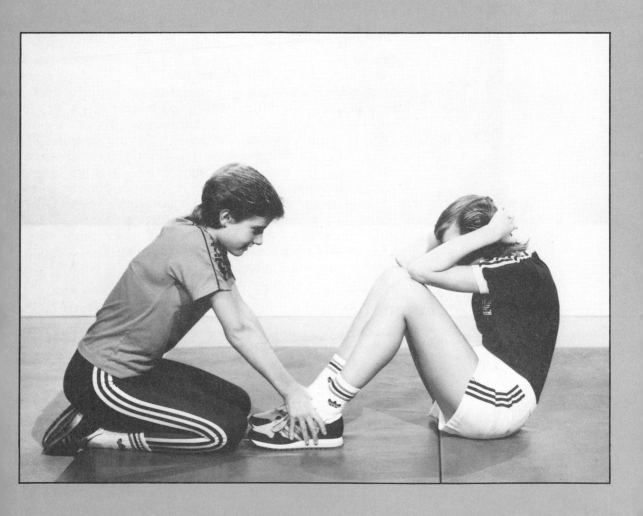

Muscular Endurance

Muscular endurance can be defined as the ability of a muscle or group of muscles to continue contracting over a period of time against a light to moderate load. A person having good muscular endurance has the capacity to work over an extended period of time without tiring quickly.

Desirably high levels of muscular endurance are usually more important in performance types of physical activities (e.g. a number of sit-ups) than in health related fitness. However, significant improvements of endurance in the more important muscle groups (e.g. upper limb muscles, anterior abdominal muscles) help reduce the risks of muscle and tendon strains even when working against a moderate load for a period of time (e.g. carrying a child or the shopping).

The terms muscular endurance and cardiovascular fitness are sometimes confused, but they are quite different. Cardiovascular fitness ensures that the heart, lungs and blood vessels work longer and more efficiently during exercise. On the other hand, good muscular endurance makes sure that the other muscles in the body do the same i.e. work longer and more efficiently during exercise. The two terms are complementary. To have good muscular endurance you do require some cardiovascular fitness. Having more than sufficient muscular endurance is extremely important to people who participate in sports like basketball, tennis, cycling and race walking. In fact, muscular endurance is more important to them than a high level of muscular strength. This presumes, of course, that they possess adequate strength.

Increasing muscular endurance

As muscular endurance influences almost all vigorous performances, methods of increasing it are important. We have discussed already the need to apply the concept of progressive overload for the development of muscular strength. This concept must be applied also if endurance is to be increased. Overload for endurance means simply working the body beyond previous endurance levels.

Development of muscular endurance

It has been established that strength contributes to muscle endurance. In fact there is a very high correlation between muscular strength and muscular endurance. Stronger individuals are usually able to continue an exercise longer than weaker ones.

Muscular endurance can be increased by any form of exercise which results in overloading the muscles, either in weight or repetitions. For example, pull-ups and bar dips, flexibility exercises, sports participation, manual labour, jogging and walking are all effective for developing endurance in the muscles in which regular overloading is accomplished. It should be noted however, that muscular endurance is highly specific. Significant increases will be limited to the muscles which experience overloading regularly. In weight training, muscular endurance is developed by performing high repetitions and low resistance.

To gain full benefit, the exercise should be similar to the activity for which you are training. The person who desires strength and endurance is advised to perform both strength exercises and endurance exercises. The principle of training specificity (i.e. strength training for strength acquisition, endurance training for increased endurance fitness) must be observed to ensure optimal development within any fitness parameter.

Muscular endurance tests

Many good tests of muscular endurance have been developed and two will be described. Try and perform these tests properly, otherwise you are only cheating yourself.

1 Sit-ups This is a test of abdominal muscle strength and endurance. The abdominals are an important muscle group in the older person. A weak or protruding stomach can cause problems such as lower back strain, and also looks unattractive.

Lie on your back with your legs together but bent at a 90° angle and clasp your hands behind your neck. A partner should hold the ankles firmly for support. Raise yourself up, using only your stomach muscles until your elbows touch your knees and then return to the starting position. This action scores one point. Repeat this action as many times as you can in one minute to score additional points. As a safety precaution, do not hold your breath during the minute of exercise.

Table 11 Abdominal muscle strength and endurance rating

	Men 35 and below	Men 36–45	Women 35 and below	Women 36–45	Boys 16–18 years	Girls 16–18 years
Excellent	48	42	40	35	46	36
Good	42	35	35	26	38	31
Average	35	26	26	19	33	23
Fair	26	18	19	15	23	17
Poor	18	12	15	12	17	14

Figure 46 Sit-ups

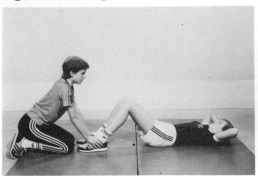 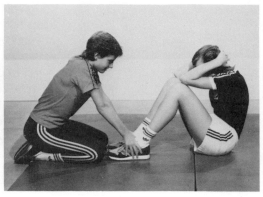

2 Circuit training This is a very special form of training which concentrates on different parts of the body and general endurance. The circuit normally consists of eight to ten exercises concentrating on the legs, abdominals, back, arms and shoulders, and trunk. The exercises should be organised so you move from one muscle group to another. This method allows you to work hard on a muscle group and then rest it, while the other groups have their turn to work out. Once all the exercises have been done, you have completed a circuit.

Although each muscle group rests in turn, at no time should the heart and lungs recover. You must go straight from one exercise station to another without stopping and you must keep each exercise going as fast as you can until the time to change.

There are many different types of circuit training. The one described below involves little apparatus and is easy to perform.

It is extremely important to first familiarise yourself with the exercises you will do. Each exercise should be performed correctly. You can determine the amount of repetitions to be performed at the stations with preliminary testing at each one. For example, if you test yourself on sit-ups and find you can perform a maximum of twenty, halve this number and set the exercise load at that station at ten. This same procedure can be carried out with the other exercises. In some, such as bench stepping, you may wish to select a workload equal to 30–60 seconds of exercise, depending on your level of fitness.

Once the first circuit is completed, rest for two or three minutes. Record the time it takes for the circuit. Your improvement will become obvious as the time required for you to complete the circuit decreases. It is also important to keep a record of your time(s), especially if you cannot make further progress. If this is so, then variation of the circuit will be needed. Such variation should be gradual and progressive.

Table 12 A fitness circuit for the beginner

Exercise	Time (depending on initial fitness)
Warm-up (see pages 3, 97)	5–10 minutes
Press-ups (Figure 64)	½ maximum
Sit-ups (Figure 46)	½ maximum
Astride jumps (Figure 47)	30/60 seconds
Lateral raise (Figure 35)	30/60 seconds
Side bends (Figure 38)	30/60 seconds
Squat thrusts (Figure 48)	½ maximum
Press behind neck (Figure 37)	30/60 seconds
Cool down (see pages 5, 99)	4–5 minutes

The advantage of circuit training is that it is possible to change the system in several different ways:

1 By performing the circuit faster
2 By increasing the number of circuits before resting
3 By decreasing the rest time between circuits
4 By increasing the number of repetitions within the circuit
5 By increasing the weight on any barbell that is used in the circuit.

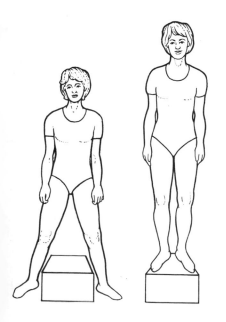

Figure 47
Astride jump over a bench

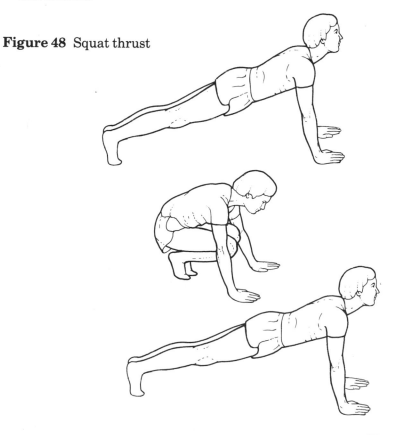

Figure 48 Squat thrust

It is extremely important to observe caution when beginning a circuit training programme. You must be fairly fit before commencing. In general, circuit training is not recommended for older people, especially for untrained sedentary individuals. It provides all round physical development, but has high intensity levels.

The following two exercises have not been covered elsewhere and are illustrated page 67 for circuit training.

Astride jump   Stand astride a bench or other suitable platform. When ready, jump with both feet to stand on the bench and then return to the starting position. Repeat this action rhythmically and continuously.

Squat thrust   From the front support position, jump with both feet to a crouch position and then jump both feet back to the front support position. Repeat this action rhythmically and continuously.

Having more than sufficient muscular endurance is extremely beneficial. It is the most significant factor in the performance of strenuous sports like rugby, soccer, swimming and basketball. In less strenuous sports such as golf, endurance is of less importance. However, even in this sport, a small amount of fatigue can influence performance adversely. Strength, timing, speed of movement, reaction time and mental alertness are all affected.

Even for those people who do not take part in sport, an adequate amount of muscular endurance is essential for daily living. The fit person has many physical and mental advantages over a person who is not as healthy. The most important physical advantage is that a person's internal organs and other body structures, such as the heart, lungs and muscles, all function better. Along with improved body function, the physically fit person enjoys a higher level of energy and finds that he or she has greater muscular strength and muscular endurance for performing daily tasks. A further advantage is that the fit person also looks healthy and vigorous. He or she has a firm, trim body, good posture, and moves well.

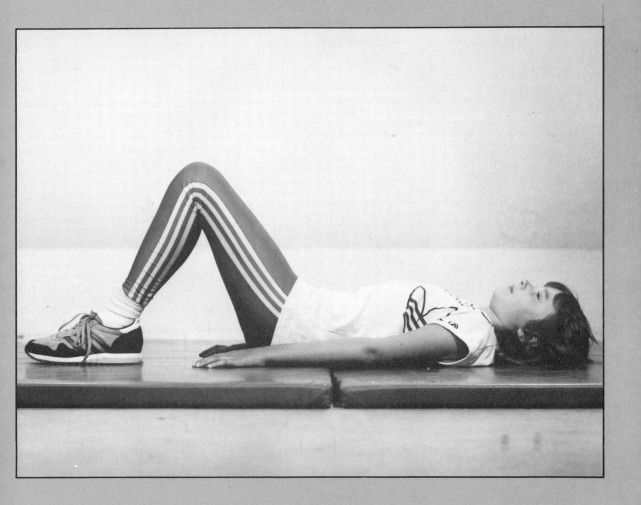

6

Stress and Relaxation

The term stress refers to the tensions and pressures which come in the wake of modern living. Economic uncertainty, traffic jams, work and unemployment can all cause stress.

People react to stress in different ways. Some people perform extremely well under stressful conditions. A limited amount of stimulation is necessary for a good performance. However, too much can give rise to anxiety, panic and even illness. Many people tend to exhibit one type of physical reaction, such as headaches, stomach upsets, respiratory problems or high blood pressure. Today, more and more people are suffering from stress. Unless combatted, stress can lead to severe health problems.

Stress sufferers

Modern daily living does not get easier. The pressures could be one of the main reasons why more and more of us show stress symptoms. These symptoms are not confined to adults. Many young people suffer from stressful conditions as well. The pressures include examinations, family problems, anxiety about acceptance by peers, problems such as anorexia nervosa, worries about physical growth and fears about unemployment.

Personality types

There is some evidence that people with certain personality traits are more prone to stress. These individuals are extremely impatient, ambitious, highly competitive and constantly working under pressure. Many people who suffer from coronary disease have this kind of Type A personality. The medical profession strongly recommends that they alter their lifestyles in order to prevent suffering from a heart attack. Exercise, as recommended throughout this book, has great potential for off-setting some of the tensions and stresses felt so intensely by Type A people.

The Type B personality is much more free of stress. These people tend to be more calm and relaxed. They accept crises philosophically. As with all attempts to categorise people, the division into Type A and Type B is slightly unrealistic. We are likely to exhibit a mixture of both patterns of behaviour. However, we should try to become more like Type B and less like Type A.

There are ways of reducing the effects of stress in your daily life. Some suggestions follow:

Hints on reducing and avoiding stress:

1 Know yourself and how much pressure *you* can handle. Try not to leave everything until the last moment. Work at a reasonable pace and avoid hurrying.

2 Take regular exercise.

3 Get away from it all when you can. Hobbies and leisure pursuits are a great help. Take a regular holiday.

4 Have enough rest and sleep. Don't start worrying about things before going to sleep.

5 When anxious or worried by events, try not to drink more than usual. The problem will still be there in the morning!

6 Endeavour to change things straight away if they are becoming a regular source of anxiety.

7 Try not to lose your temper. Control your feelings if possible.

8 Eat meals slowly and don't think of work or problems while eating.

9 Don't be competitive all of the time. The strain will catch up with you, especially when you get older.

10 Relax the muscles with some deep breathing.

Make an attempt to avoid creating stressful conditions for yourself. Absence of stress improves the quality of life, and even its length!

Relaxation

You are never too busy to relax for at least a short while each day. Relaxation can improve your efficiency at work and play, increase your energy and drive. This will generally benefit your health and happiness. Fatigue and aches caused by prolonged muscle tension are eliminated, good sleeping habits are encouraged and pain can be more easily tolerated through relaxation.

Relaxation is of vital importance but it is of no benefit if you relax with a guilty conscience. Children should be taught relaxation as part of their physical education programme. It is a preventive measure against the anxiety that often occurs in adult life. Relaxation is not a cure for conditions that require medical treatment, although it can help them. Nor can relaxation remove personal or occupational problems. However, relaxation diminishes your reaction to problems which can be the first step towards solving them.

Relaxation techniques

It is no good telling some people to relax because they have nurtured a habit of muscle tension over the years and cannot recognise these inappropriate contractions as such. To prevent yourself reaching this state you must first of all learn to recognise tension.

1 Feeling tension by touch

An effective way of finding out whether your muscles are tensed is by touch. You will be able to tell the difference between a tense, contracted muscle and a soft resting one, either on yourself or a partner. Let us use the example of the arm.

With your left hand reach across and take hold of the top of your right upper arm. Lift the right arm slightly. It will now be tense. Touch it all over. Now let your arm relax by your side and feel the difference.

Perform this test action again, but without actually lifting your right arm. Just prepare to do so. You will feel a different degree of tension this time. This type of contraction occurs when you are prepared for action. Release the tension and feel the difference. We can now appreciate the difference regarding bodily movement and muscle tension.

2 Learning through observation

This is another way of recognising tension. Observe movement in other people as they perform physical activities. Look out for the tense and relaxed phases of the movement.

The majority of top athletes exhibit ease of movement in their performances. This is a result of an economy of effort with muscles contracting only when they are required to.

Look out as well for tenseness in other people. Hunched shoulders and nail-biting are examples of tense behaviour. Some people are tense even when they are asleep.

3 Learning by contrasting contraction and relaxation of muscles

This technique was developed by Dr Edmund Jacobson in the USA. Its aim is to concentrate on a strong contraction of the muscles and then feel the relaxation as the tension is released. The whole of the body is involved and it takes a little time to master the technique. A programme which can be used by children and adults is given in *Table 13*.

4 Biofeedback instruments

This technique involves making a reading from an instrument of physiological reactions that result from nervousness and tension. Examples of such reactions are increased pulse rate, increased sweating and muscle tension. Temperature changes can be measured also if you have a simple instrument available. This method can be useful for learning relaxation techniques.

When a person becomes more or less nervous, there are corresponding changes in the electrical resistance of the

Table 13 Relaxation programme (contraction–relaxation)

Part of body	Time	Action/feelings
Arms	5 mins	i Contract your fingers to make a fist. Relax. Notice the difference when relaxed. ii Bend your elbows and tense your biceps. Relax. Notice the relaxed feeling of your muscles.
Facial area	5 mins	i Make a face; wrinkle your forehead and nose. Relax. Notice how pleasant the relaxation feels. ii Clench your jaws, bite your teeth together. Relax. Appreciate the relaxation. iii Press your tongue hard against the roof of your mouth. Relax. Notice the difference.
Shoulders and upper back	5 mins	i Raise shoulders as high as possible in the sitting position for a few minutes. Relax. Notice the relaxation.
Chest, stomach and lower back	5 mins	i Relax the body. Breathe in and out freely. Notice that relaxation increases as you exhale. ii Make your stomach hard for as long as possible. Relax. Notice the difference when the stomach is properly relaxed.
Thighs and buttocks	3 mins	i Tense your buttocks as firmly as possible. Relax.
Calves	2 mins	i *Dorsi-flex* the foot (pull insteps and toes towards shin). Relax. Notice the difference between the tension and relaxation.

skin. This is due to a change in the amount of sweating. You can learn to control these reactions. Instruments are available that register such changes. The advantage in using them lies in the fact that they will register clearly and accurately whether relaxation has been effective, and to what degree.

5 Breathing, yoga and meditation

Controlled breathing has been employed by many oriental religions for several thousands of years as part of the meditative process. Meditation involves concentrating on breathing for long periods without distraction. It is part of the search for total relaxation.

Hatha yoga concerns itself with physical health and incorporates the practice of various postures accompanied by controlled breathing and relaxation. This postural practice clearly increases flexibility and bodily control. Concentration on breathing helps to achieve better mental relaxation.

6 Massage   Massage stimulates the flow of blood and improves muscle tone. It assists in the clearing away of waste products and in the reduction of muscular tension and associated pain.

However, it also does more than this. During massage there is a gentle calming down of the whole body without concentrating the mind. Massage offers recuperative rest from everyday stress.

There are many different ways to find relaxation and calmness of mind. What may be successful for one person in a particular environment may not be suitable for someone else who has a different physical and mental make-up. Prayer, yoga, meditation and other forms of relaxation techniques are methods which have helped numerous people. Whatever method you use, it must be practised regularly until it becomes a habit in your daily life. This will help you achieve the best results. The aim should be not to become a recluse and withdraw from the world but to build up resources so that you can cope with stress without distress.

One of the most effective means of coping with stress is through regular physical activity, as outlined in this book. Appropriate leisure pursuits which include proper exercise provide a successful way of managing the ever growing problems of stress in today's society.

Figure 49 Neck and shoulder massage

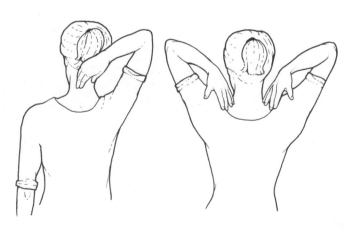

Gentle massage of the neck and shoulder region relieves tightness and improves circulation.

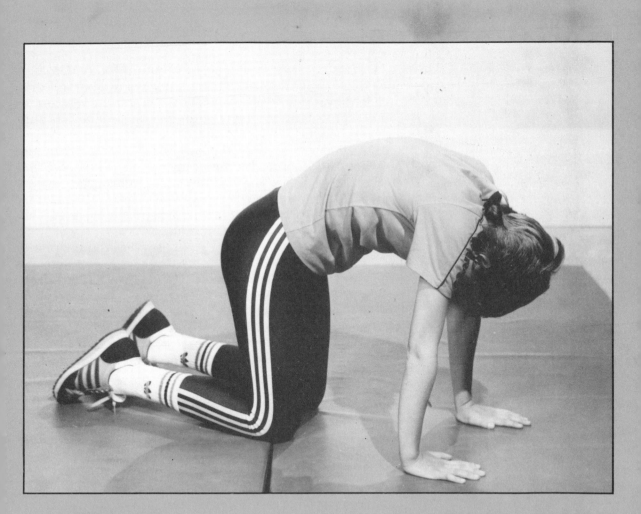

7

Additional Considerations

If you are healthy and fit, you considerably reduce your chances of ever suffering from hypokinetic diseases or conditions. These are caused in part by a lack of physical activity. In fact, the term hypokinetic (first used by Kraus and Raab in 1961) means too little exercise or less than acceptable energy expenditure. Such diseases include heart trouble, high blood pressure, pain in the lower back and obesity. It is generally the middle-aged and elderly who are prone to these problems but they can start to develop during youth. Therefore, the younger age group in particular needs education for health related fitness.

Posture

1 Lower back pain and postural problems

Back ache affects many people in Britain today. On any one day, approximately 88,000 adults are unable to work due to lower back problems. This costs the nation a considerable sum of money through lost production and sickness benefit.

In the majority of cases, the lower back ache is due to the fact that the structures in the spinal region do not have the strength to support the body weight. Appropriate exercises correctly performed can alleviate this problem. It is extremely important to have sufficient strength in the muscles of the back and abdominals.

Good posture habits should be observed and exercises for the back practised every day so that back problems do not occur. Postural problems start early in life and need constant attention by all.

Many children have similar postures to their parents. This is due to heredity as well as imitation. Height is another factor which influences posture. For example, short individuals tend to stand very upright whilst tall individuals often stoop slightly, rounding their backs and necks.

There appears to be a strong relationship between posture and such things as perceptual acuity, emotional health, and general fitness. Chronic television viewing and inadequate daily exercise produce numerous postural problems. These are readily detectable and can be corrected by exercise, particularly at an early age.

There is no clear definition or standard of 'good' posture that can be applied to all people whether they are standing, sitting or moving. Standing posture is judged by the alignment of body segments. Figure 50 illustrates good posture because the body segments are evenly balanced over the base of support. Viewed from the side, the plumb line runs from a little in front of the ankle through the knee, pelvis, shoulders and ear. In this position the

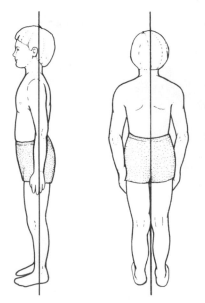

Figure 50 Good posture (side and back view)

natural curves of the body are moderate, with the head, shoulders, pelvis, knees and feet balanced evenly on each side of the line. Viewed from the back, the plumb line runs midway through the head, vertebrae, and hips and is equidistant between the feet.

A person with good posture requires a minimum contraction of antigravity muscle groups to keep his or her body erect and balanced. However, when a person slouches, his or her upper back muscles must contract to shift the body to the correct posture. If he or she continues to slouch, the muscles will gradually adapt to that position. Eventually he or she will have chronic poor posture if the poor posture is not corrected.

Common posture problems

With proper exercise, particularly if started at an early age, many typical posture deviations can be corrected. The following deviations can be observed when the individual is standing beside a plumb line:

Round upper back (kyphosis)

Round upper back, or kyphosis, is characterised by a marked increase in the curve of the upper back (**Figure 51**). The head and shoulders are usually held in a forward position, and the backward curve of the upper body causes the pelvis to tilt forward slightly and the knees to bend somewhat. This condition puts more strain on the upper back muscles and shifts the weight of the body to the front of the foot.

Hollow back (lordosis)

Hollow back, or lordosis, is an exaggerated forward curve of the lower back (**Figure 52**). The most common signs are a protruding abdomen and hyperextension of the knees.

Figure 51 Round upper back (kyphosis)

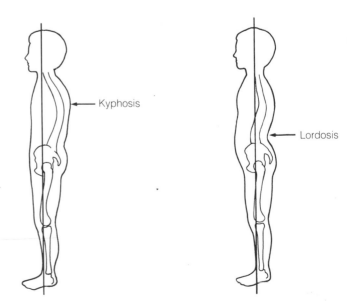

Figure 52 Hollow back (lordosis)

/ *Lateral curvature (scoliosis)*

Lateral curvature, or scoliosis, can be C-shaped (extending the length of the spinal column) or S-shaped (with a small curve on the upper back and a compensating curve on the lower back). (*See* **Figure 53**.)

The C-shaped curve is normally toward the left since most people are right handed and tend to lean to the weaker side. This comes from the constant elevation of the right arm and the tendency to lean toward the left side of the desk/office table while writing and performing other activities while sitting. The S-shaped curvature develops over a period of time from such poor postural body positions as holding one shoulder higher than the other, head tilting to one side, hips not level and body weight carried more by one leg than the other. Early attention to lateral curvature is important because it generally gets worse instead of better with age.

Figure 53 Lateral curvature (scoliosis)

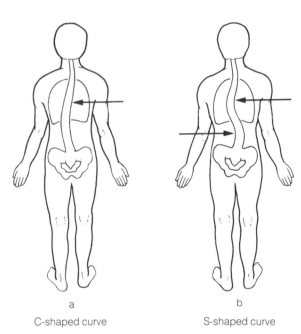

a
C-shaped curve

b
S-shaped curve

Methods of assessing posture in school children

The Physical Education teacher is generally in the best position to assess the postures of pupils. Most PE teachers are genuinely concerned about the way children sit, stand and move in their daily activities. The evaluation of posture is primarily one of continual subjective observation. When a teacher notices a major change in a child's posture, the teacher should contact the school nurse or doctor or parent. It is important to determine whether the change is due to a muscular weakness or to other factors, such as poor nutrition, poor eyesight, or an emotional disturbance.

If a PE teacher wishes to use a simple screening test, he or she might consider the side and rear view plumb line test and the posture chart shown in *Table 14*. The chart can be used in various ways, depending on the interests of the teacher, the ages of the children and the time available. The test can be completed in the classroom.

Methods of improving posture

The plumb line test is designed as a basic screening device. It can detect major postural problems and, perhaps more importantly, make the child more conscious of his or her posture when standing, sitting or moving. The foundation of good posture, however, is the possession of optimum levels of muscular strength, endurance, flexibility, and efficient motor skill patterns. The following exercises will assist in correcting functional postural defects. These exercises also improve general muscular strength, endurance and flexibility.

1 Exercises for improving round shoulders

Hanging (**Figure 54**) Hang from a horizontal bar, or wall bars, facing outwards with feet just off the floor.

Wall push (**Figure 55**) Stand about two feet from a wall with palms touching it at shoulder height. Keeping the body straight, bend your elbows until the chest almost touches the wall, then return to the starting position.

Head and arm raise (**Figure 56**) Lie face downwards with forehead resting on your hands, arms bent. Raise head, hands and elbows about 6 cm. Keep head and hands in this position but continue raising elbows as high as possible.

Figure 54 Hanging (strength and endurance)

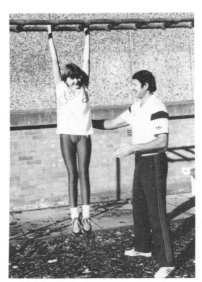

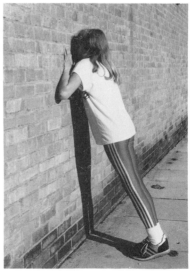

Figure 55 Wall push (strength and flexibility)

Figure 56 Head and arm raise (strength and flexibility)

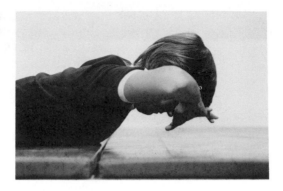

2 Exercises for improving lower back

Cat stretcher (**Figure 57**) Start in a partially crouched position and then stretch back upwards. Hold at the highest point for a few seconds and then return to the starting position.

Flexion of vertebral column (**Figure 58**) Lie on your back with legs bent and knees held by the arms. Move the knees towards the chest to lengthen the long spinal muscles and shorten the abdominals.

Hollow back pressing (**Figure 60**) Lie on your back with legs bent. Press the hollow of the back against the floor.

The exercises in **Figures 57–60** will also help older people to improve and strengthen muscles of the body which ensure good posture.

Figure 57 Cat stretcher (strength and flexibility)

Figure 58 Flexion of vertebral column (strength and flexibility)

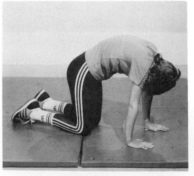
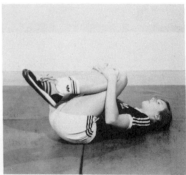

Perhaps the most obvious reason for obtaining good posture is that it makes you look better. Everyone wants to look good. Remember, the first impression you make upon a stranger is visual! Another reason for having good posture is that your body will be more efficient. Joints, ligaments and muscles will not be incorrectly strained and your range of movement will be greater. Postural faults are linked to poor health. Lordosis tends to make one more susceptible to backache. Kyphosis may impair respiratory capacity. Scoliosis can result in serious deformity and a painful back if not treated early.

Figure 59 Posture (side and back view)

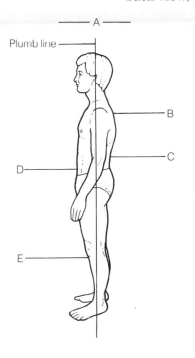

Table 14 A Posture chart, using a Plumb Line

Name _____

Date _____

Evaluation 1 _____

Evaluation 2 _____

Evaluation 3 _____

Score:-
   Correct   0
   Fair   1
   Poor   2

Note: Use figure 59a and 59b as correct (0) rating.

	Side view	Evaluation 1	Evaluation 2	Evaluation 3
A	Body Lean: Forward			
	Backward			
B	Round shoulders			
C	Hollow back			
D	Protruding abdomen			
E	Knees forced back			
	Back view			
F	Shoulder: dropped on right			
	dropped on left			
G	Curve of vertebrae: C-curve			
	S-curve			
H	Bow legs			
I	Knock knees			
J	Feet: pointing out			
	pointing in			

Another safeguard for the back (particularly for older people) is to make sure that you lift weights or objects with your legs bent, keeping your back straight. Getting close to the weight or object being lifted will ease the enormous strain on the lower back.

Remember to keep your back straight when doing household chores such as the washing-up or making the bed. You only have one back, so make doubly sure that you look after it during your lifetime. Once injured, you will have a weakness and it might result in lower back pain later in life.

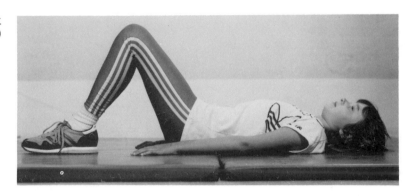

Figure 60 Hollow back pressing (strength)

2 Coronary heart disease

One of the greatest epidemics that we have experienced in recent years is coronary heart disease. It is a disease associated with a number of factors such as fat, stress and smoking. Heart disease kills about 180,000 people in Britain each year.

What happens is that one of the arteries in the heart muscle is narrowed by atherosclerosis. This occurs when fatty substances such as cholesterol are deposited beneath the lining of the arteries, forming plaques. The result is that blood circulation is reduced to that area. The probability of a heart attack will be greater. If a person is fit, he or she has a greater chance of recovering from such an attack.

Coronary heart disease can start to develop during childhood as habits and lifestyle are learned at an early age. It is therefore important for physical educators and others concerned with young people to attempt to minimise the risks of cardiovascular disease. Research findings from both the UK and USA reveal that coronary heart disease can be reduced if we smoke less, lower our fat intake and increase our level of physical activity. A strong healthy heart is able to cope better in times of stress and can function more effectively and efficiently. However, there is still some disagreement among medical

Figure 61 Right and wrong
ways of lifting objects

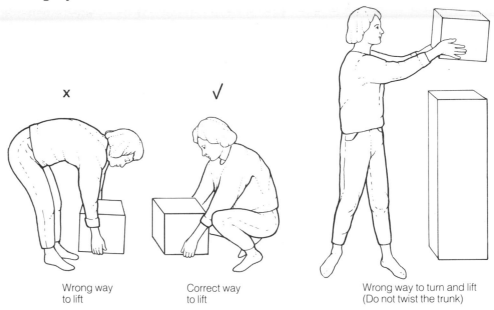

Wrong way
to lift

Correct way
to lift

Wrong way to turn and lift
(Do not twist the trunk)

authorities as to the causes of this disease and the best
preventive measures.

3 High blood pressure (hypertension)

Medical evidence suggests that the condition known as
high blood pressure (hypertension) greatly increases your
risk of heart trouble and other serious illnesses.

In simple terms, blood pressure is the force that the
blood exerts against the blood vessel walls. Pressure is
present in all types of blood vessels but arterial blood
pressure is the one most commonly measured and most
important to our health. Systolic blood pressure represents the phase during which the heart is pumping blood
through the arterial system. Pressure is then greatest
against the arterial wall. Increases in the amount of blood
being pumped from the heart can increase the systolic
blood pressure. The diastolic blood pressure is that which
exists when the heart is resting i.e. between the beats.

A number of factors influence the normal range of blood
pressure. These factors include age, body position (such as
sitting or standing), time of day, level of exercise, and
intake of caffeine, alcohol and nicotine. There is a rather
wide range in blood pressure levels, both systolic and
diastolic, from one individual to another. For example, at
age twenty the range is about 90–145 for systolic and
50–95 for diastolic. A level of 140 for systolic and 90 for
diastolic is considered to be hypertension. Some twenty-
year-olds have high blood pressure. As age increases, the
upper ranges of both systolic and diastolic pressures in-

crease also. A greater proportion of older people become hypertensive. A persistent resting blood pressure of over 140 systolic and/or 90 diastolic is considered high. The person is in need of medical help and attention. High blood pressure can be controlled to some extent by modern drugs prescribed by doctors.

Figure 62 Normal and high blood pressure

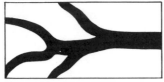

Normal blood pressure

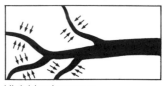

High blood pressure

Steps to take to reduce or avoid high blood pressure

There is a lot that you can do to help keep your blood pressure at a normal level, or reduce it if it is high. These measures are as follows:

1 Reduce body weight if overweight.
2 Avoid unnecessary stress both at home and work.
3 Eat foods that are good for health. Cut out high fat foods and substitute lean meat, chicken and poultry.
4 Eat less salt.
5 Give up smoking.
6 Take exercise on a regular basis.
7 If you are over 35, have your blood pressure tested regularly.

4 Smoking

Widespread evidence suggests that cigarette smoking, even in moderation, is deleterious to the health. Britain has one of the highest death rates in the world from lung cancer and much of this has been associated with smoking. Smoking is not usually considered a childhood problem although there is concern about young people taking up the habit. It is during adolescence that the addiction to cigarettes is often formed.

Nicotine has a depressant action on the appetite and the smoke irritates the membrane lining the respiratory passages. This can give rise to chronic bronchitis, shortness of breath and smokers' cough. Other physiological effects include the increased likelihood of lung cancer and heart disease in later life. Women who smoke while pregnant risk retarding the growth of their unborn children and making them more susceptible to respiratory diseases.

Excessive smoking is often associated with other undesirable habits such as the failure to take regular or adequate meals and failure to get sufficient sleep. The use of tobacco is sometimes supposed to be a cure for 'nervousness' but, far from being a sedative, it may encourage nervous signs and symptoms.

There is no evidence that smoking does any good for anyone. There is much evidence that it is harmful. Therefore, it is desirable for all of us not to smoke. In addition, there are social disadvantages to the habit. The smell and discolouration of teeth which result are not attractive. The medical profession and the Health Education Council have shown that it is never too late to give up or cut down on smoking.

Needless to say, smoking is incompatible with a healthy lifestyle. If you do not smoke now, resolve never to start. If you are a smoker and want to improve your health, you must want to stop.

The following suggestions may help you to give up smoking:

1 Gradually reduce the number of cigarettes you smoke per day to reach a deadline for giving up altogether.

2 If possible, encourage a friend to stop with you. You can help each other.

3 Join a stop smoking programme.

4 Use one of the 'stop-smoking' products on the market.

5 Think of smoking as the expensive and dirty habit that it is.

6 Be strong-willed and think of other things to do.

7 Always remember that smoking can cause serious illness.

8 Contact the Health Education Council for advice.

5 Alcohol

Alcohol is a drug and a potent depressant that may exert harmful effects on the human body if consumed in excessive amounts. In moderation, alcohol consumption appears not to be detrimental to your health. Moderate drinking is interpreted as no more than 1–2 pints of beer or two glasses of wine per day. For some individuals, moderate drinking can be beneficial. A drink or two may serve as a relaxant and a stress reducer. For people who are dieting to lose weight, however, the additional calories in alcohol will make weight loss more difficult.

Health problems of a serious nature are associated with chronic excessive drinking. The acute effects include impairment of both motor co-ordination and judgement. These are factors extremely important in the safe control and operation of a car. Drunken driving is the cause of many deaths in Britain today. Excessive alcoholic drinking is also a major cause of many household accidents and family abuse.

Over a period of years, chronic consumption of excessive amounts of alcohol may have detrimental effects on various body organs, particularly the liver. The liver begins to accumulate fatty deposits. The liver cells degenerate eventually and are replaced by non-functioning scar tissue. This condition is known as cirrhosis. Many of the social problems associated with smoking apply also to excessive drinking. There are the bad effects on appearance and behaviour, as well as the unnecessary expense.

The immediate effects of excessive alcohol on a person depend upon a number of different factors, such as body size, amount of food in the stomach and the individual's state of mind. In general, however, the following symptoms are typical:

Number of pints of beer consumed in one night	Typical effects
1–2	Reduced tension; relief from daily stress
3–5	Co-ordination and fine motor ability impaired
6–8	Gross motor co-ordination impaired; staggering gait
9–10	Loss of control of voluntary motor ability; sleep or dazed feeling
11 and above	Coma; depression of respiratory centres

The following are some general recommendations for making alcoholic drink part of a healthy lifestyle:

1 Drink moderately and infrequently, or not at all.

2 Know your capacity and do not exceed it.

3 Eat some food, particularly some protein and fat, before or while you drink.

4 Drink slowly. Do not gulp.

5 Don't drink to solve a problem. The problem will be there in the morning.

6 Do not drink alcohol if you are taking other drugs that may also be depressants or cause drowsiness.

7 Do not drive after drinking, and do not let your friends do so either. Go by public transport or hire a taxi.

8 Get medical or professional help (e.g. Alcoholics Anonymous) if you have a problem with alcohol.

Remember, those who never drink and those who drink in moderation can enjoy the same level of good health.

6 Exercise cautions

It is extremely important to follow guidelines when taking part in physical activity or sport. In earlier sections, certain cautions were discussed relating to exercises for cardiovascular fitness, flexibility, muscular strength and muscular endurance.

For example, if we perform too much exercise too soon it can result in poor recovery between training sessions. This causes a poorer performance, a decreased work capacity and a loss of enjoyment and motivation. If these problems occur, it is advisable to diminish the intensity, frequency or duration of your physical activity programme.

There are danger signs which indicate that exercise must be stopped immediately. These are:

a Laboured breathing (i.e. difficult breathing, not the deep breathing normally associated with exercise)

b Loss of co-ordination

c Dizziness

d Tightness in chest.

If any of the above occurs, exercise should be discontinued until medical advice is obtained.

If you act as a leader of an exercise programme, you should always:

a Be alert for signs of too fast a pace.

b Watch for signs of over-exertion.

c Caution participants to resist competitive urges which lead to over-stress.

d Maintain a friendly, jovial climate for the class.

e Be prepared to adjust the workout to accommodate daily and seasonal differences in temperature and humidity.

f Maintain records. The leader is responsible for the progress of the participants.

Ultimately it is up to you as leader to judge the ability of the class to progress from one stage to the next. You should know your class and be responsible for it.

A physical fitness leader should be knowledgeable about the prevention and care of injuries associated with exercise, but not to the extent of assuming the role of a medical doctor. Simple preventive measures, advice and injury care given at the right time can mean the difference between continued participation and temporary incapacitation.

There are a few exercises used today that can cause injury and joint damage. These include the toe touching exercise, straight leg sit-ups, hurdler's stretch, the knees stretch and the forced back hyperextension. Pain or injury might not be felt straight away. Sometimes the damage is gradual and will not appear until later on in life.

Many young people today are given demanding training programmes that undoubtedly will affect a proportion of them when they get older. Some young people drop out of these programmes. One probable cause may be the fact that a large number of participants are injured as a result of physical activity. Other young people lose interest because they have unhappy memories or experiences, some of which occur through excess physical and psychological stress. This is happening at a time when they are either physically or mentally not up to facing such stress because of their age.

As mentioned earlier, training programmes are becoming increasingly more demanding for the talented individual. For example, a good school soccer player aged about 14 probably trains three times weekly and plays two games of soccer. If he or she is a good all-rounder, he or she may represent the school in another sport as well. Such a schedule would be demanding enough for an adult, let alone a growing teenager.

Over-use injuries in the form of bone pains, particularly in young soccer players, are becoming well known. An example is Osgood Schlatter's disease. This involves swelling and tenderness over the knob below the kneecap. The disease occurs only in growing children.

We also need to be aware of the playing and training surface because stress fractures can result if they are poor and hard.

As long as we are aware of the 'over-use' syndrome, then the chances of our students receiving damaging injuries now and later on in life will be lessened. Perhaps a monitoring system should be introduced to negate the incidence of stress and over-use injuries.

As teachers, coaches and leaders we must always, remember the negative effects which can result if insufficient care is taken.

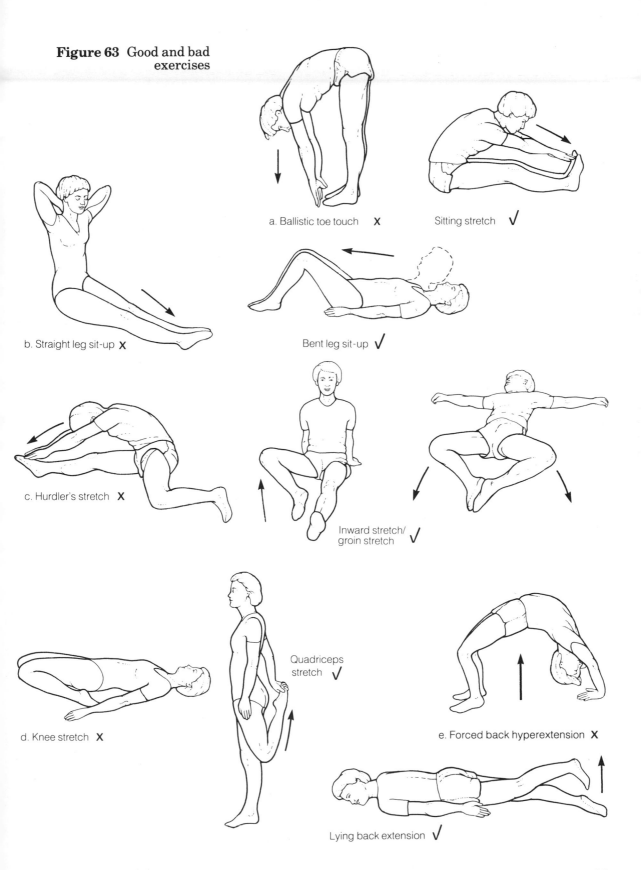

Figure 63 Good and bad exercises

a. Ballistic toe touch **X**

Sitting stretch **√**

b. Straight leg sit-up **X**

Bent leg sit-up **√**

c. Hurdler's stretch **X**

Inward stretch/ groin stretch **√**

d. Knee stretch **X**

Quadriceps stretch **√**

e. Forced back hyperextension **X**

Lying back extension **√**

7 Exercise and pregnancy

There is no reason why you should stop being active during pregnancy. Exercise during this period and after giving birth is as essential to good health as under ordinary circumstances. With regular exercise, you will not only feel better but also be better prepared for the delivery of your baby. Many daily activities such as sitting, standing, walking, stair climbing, kneeling and squatting are good forms of exercise. Since these activities compose a much greater percentage of your movements during the day than a regular exercise routine, they should be performed with efficient body mechanics. Women who have a background of sports participation or who are habitually active tend to have fewer complications during pregnancy as well as quicker and easier deliveries. This is because of their good cardiovascular system, muscle control and abdominal muscle tone. Women who possess a high degree of physiological fitness appear to be bothered less with common gynaecological problems than women who are unfit.

However, beginning a programme of physical activity at the onset of pregnancy might be unwise. A 'crash' course of physical activity during pregnancy does not produce the benefits derived from such activity pursued over a long period of time. If you choose to begin a programme for the first time when pregnant, it is highly advisable to consult your doctor.

There are of course other considerations for health related fitness. For example, there is the problem of drug abuse, but that is beyond the scope of this book.

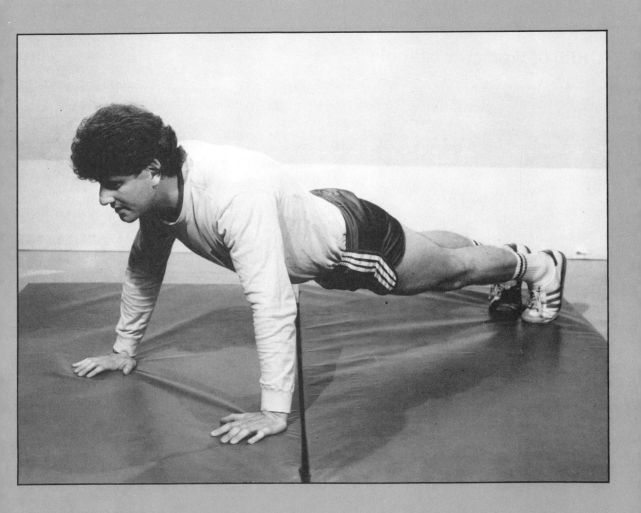

8

Scheme of Work

Concern about health and fitness is growing amongst the general public but actual knowledge and development of the right habits are lagging behind. As a result, there is a need to provide our pupils in schools with the chance to perform both practical and theoretical aspects of health related fitness. The habits may then continue throughout their adult life.

The programme described here is for 4th and 5th year co-educational students and is both theoretical and practical in nature. Each unit is presented as a 10 week block with two 50 minute periods per week.

Units of work for schools

Health related fitness (Unit One) 4th year	(Guidelines with kind permission from Rawlins Upper School and Community College, Leicestershire)
Introduction	The importance of exercise and fitness for disease prevention. Other benefits include looking good, feeling good, and enjoying life to the full.
Physical fitness	Define cardiovascular fitness, strength and muscular endurance, flexibility, body composition, and self evaluation (all components).
Preparing for exercise	Use of proper footwear and clothing; warm-up and cool-down; gradual progression; injury prevention.
Principles of training	Adaptation; overload; specificity; individual response; use and disuse.
How to exercise	Aerobics; calisthenics; weight training; isometric exercises; stretching exercises; anaerobic exercises; gymnastic conditioning.
Accidents, first aid, safety (Unit Two) 4th year	
Introduction	Principles of first aid; how to handle an accident; bleeding; shock and fainting.
Anatomy	The skeleton; broken bones.
Physiology	Joint and muscle injuries; cramp.
Breathing	How we breathe; resuscitation; checking circulation; choking; suffocation.
Poisons and burns	Insect bites; snake bites; treating burns and scalds; sunburn; blisters from rubbing.

Unconsciousness	Nervous system; head injuries; epilepsy.
Effects of temperature	Hypothermia; frostbite; heat exhaustion; heat stroke.
Movement of casualties	Preparing a stretcher; loading a stretcher; four-handed seat; help to walk; moving a casualty to safety.
Accident scene	Role play.

Lifestyle management (Unit Three) 5th year

Introduction	What is preventative medicine?
Diet and nutrition	Role of nutrition in diet; food and drink; individual diet sheets for a week (discuss results – good/bad); health foods/supplements; myths and misconceptions; exercise and appetite.
Weight control	Energy intake and expenditure; energy balance; diets to avoid; diets to consider; change your lifestyle – exercise benefits; determining body composition.
Care of back and posture	Costs to nation and to individual; postural defects; strengthen muscles.
Stress and relaxation	What are stress and relaxation; environmental stress (e.g. demand from work); psychological stress (e.g. family death); physiological stress (e.g. body injury).

Lifestyle management (Unit Four) 5th year

Exercise cautions	High risk for injury; over-use syndrome.
Smoking	Why it is bad; display scientific results; how to stop.
Alcohol	Moderation; problems of excessive drinking.
Leisure time	Questionnaires; problems – how solved? sports clubs and leisure facilities in the community; links with local sports council.
Lifestyle problem-solving	An appraisal of individual lifestyle patterns.
Enjoying health related fitness	Positive attitude; learning new skills can be enjoyable; variety; do your own thing.

Throughout programmes in the 4th and 5th years there should be individual records of height, weight and skin-fold measurements. Fitness evaluations should take place as well.

Time to commence

With today's sedentary and automated lifestyle, none of us can take good health and fitness for granted. The way to ensure a lifetime of physical well-being is through regular exercise and developing healthy living habits. These should commence at an early age.

Now is the time to take up sports and recreational pursuits in which you can continue to participate over the years to come. Being fit and healthy brings many benefits, including improvements in your:

1 physical and mental energy
2 sleeping patterns
3 physical appearance
4 ability to relax
5 enjoyment of life
6 physical well being with a lower risk of hypokinetic disease.

The programme outlined is not meant to be regarded as either ideal or complete. It simply suggests ideas that could be followed. This means making some radical changes in our traditionally sports-based programmes in schools. Physical education can make a vital contribution towards promoting optimal health related fitness benefit through a relevant curriculum. An approach has been suggested and now it is up to you.

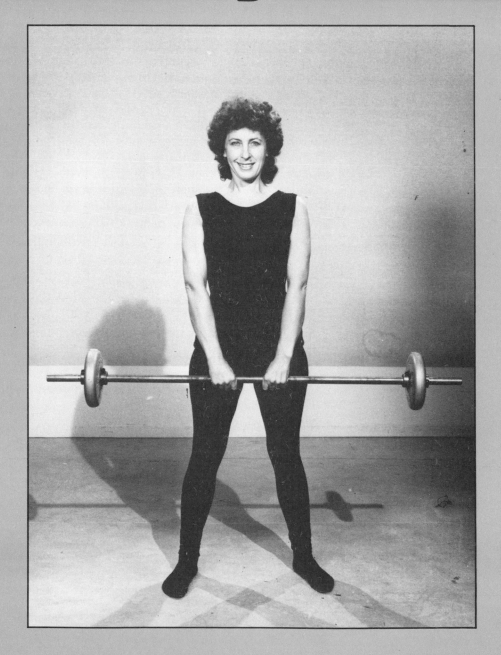

9

Adult Beginners

A considerable amount of information, and descriptions of techniques relating to health related fitness have been provided in the previous sections. You will now realise that a good diet and a properly designed exercise programme are effective ways of helping to prevent hypokinetic diseases, thus improving your chances for an increased life expectancy. In addition, you have been informed that a positive healthy lifestyle may confer immediate benefits such as improved fitness, a sense of well-being and a reduction of stressful symptoms.

Living a sedentary life and eating unwisely increases the chances of premature physiological deterioration. However, we can minimize the physiological ageing process by adapting a positive approach to health and fitness.

Make a personal commitment today. Your body and mind will thank you in later years. If you have been inactive for a number of years or have been seriously ill then get medical advice before you embark on an exercise programme.

Planning an exercise programme: some guidelines

Your exercise programme should consist of four basic components, namely:

1 The warm-up
2 Muscular strength and endurance development
3 Cardiovascular work
4 The cool-down.

It is recommended that you exercise for 40–45 minutes three times a week to gain the full rewards of the programme.

A ten week exercise programme is presented on *Table 15*. The exercises should be chosen to develop strength and muscular endurance, flexibility and cardiovascular endurance. In the early stages of the programme, there is a greater amount of time devoted to warm-up than there is later on. For the development of cardiovascular endurance, the opposite is true. This is because an allowance is made for the generally expected poor condition of the beginner. In the first few weeks, basic warm up exercises are stressful enough to help produce a cardiovascular training effect.

Strength and muscular endurance exercises are provided as an extension of the warm-up period. A few more strenuous stretching exercises are included also within the strength – endurance exercise time allocation.

For the press up, lower your body to the floor by bending your arms, keeping the body straight. Then push up to the starting position as shown in **Figure 64a**. The modified press up (**Figure 64b**) is an easier variation. The following guidelines regarding the four parts of an exercise programme should be observed by the beginner.

Table 15 Weekly progressions for beginner's programme

	Muscular strength and endurance						Cardiovascular training		
Week	Warm-up (min.)	Press ups[1]	Astride jumps	Arm/leg-lift (each side)	Sit-ups	Squat thrusts	Jogging[2]	Cool down (mins)	Total time (mins)
1	15	6M	8	5	6	6	3 × 1 min. sets	10	40
2	15	8M	9	6	7	6	3 × 1½ min. sets	10	40
3	14	10M	9	6	8	10	3 × 2 min. sets	9	41
4	14	6	10	7	9	10	3 × 2½ min. sets	9	41
5	13	7	10	7	10	15	3 × 3 min. sets	8	42
6	12	7	10	7	11	15	3 × 3½ min. sets	7	43
7	12	8	11	8	12	20	3 × 4 min. sets	7	43
8	11	8	11	8	13	20	3 × 4½ min. sets	6	44
9	10	9	12	9	14	25	3 × 25 min. sets	6	44
10	10	10	12	10	15	25	10 min. (1500m)	5	45

[1] M = modified press up
[2] A set consists of the time given for jogging followed by 2 mins recovery.

Figure 64 The press-up and the modified press-up

a. Press up   b. Modified press up

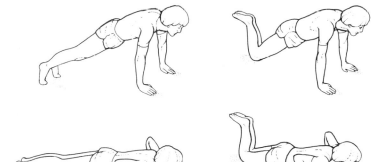

1 The Warm-up a There should be a gradual increase in the intensity of exercise as the warm-up progresses.

b The warm-up should include exercises that stretch the muscles and joints through their full range of movement. Use non-resistance exercises.

c The exercises should be performed rhythmically and flow naturally from one to another.

d Include a variety of warm-up exercises on different days. It will be more interesting and more enjoyable.

e At the beginning of your fitness programme the warm-up should last about 20 minutes. As you get fitter, the warm-up time will necessarily decrease, as the other parts of the fitness programme take more time.

f It is important that the exercises involve the circulatory system, the activity of the heart and the slow stretching of the muscles and joints.

2 Muscular strength and endurance development

a Perform all exercises through the full range of movement.

b Plan your exercises so that different parts of the body are worked in sequence (i.e. do not work any one part of the body in consecutive exercises).

c It is better to perform resistance exercises in sets rather than continuously to exhaustion. (For example, if the target of a moderately conditioned individual is to do 10 press ups it is better to perform two sets of 5 rather than one set of 10).

Suitable exercises for muscular strength and endurance development include the following:

1 Press ups (**Figure 64**) arms/shoulders

2 Astride jumps (**Figure 47**) legs

3 Arm/leg lift (**Figure 21**) back

4 Sit-ups (**Figure 40/46**) abdominals

5 Squat thrusts (**Figure 48**) arm/legs

3 Cardiovascular work

a Workout at your cardiovascular fitness level. The key is to begin slowly, gradually increasing the exercise intensity as you become better conditioned. (See *Table 15* for progression advice.)

b If you have been inactive for some time, you should begin with a less vigorous activity such as walking.

c Exercise intensity along with duration and frequency are key factors in developing cardiovascular fitness.

d As the body begins to adapt to the exercise routine over the weeks, the intensity, duration, and/or frequency may be increased.

e The following points should be observed when performing your jogging programme:

1 Simply jog in a way that is natural to you.

2 Do not try and copy anyone else's style. Joggers come in all shapes and sizes. Let your body be its own master.

3 Avoid clenching your fists, as this will cause tension in the neck and shoulders.

4 The pace should be easy and relaxed enough to be able to carry on a conversation.

5 Do not be afraid to walk if necessary. Jogging should be enjoyable and not a self-inflicted ordeal!

6 It is best to jog at the same time every day so that you can establish a daily routine. However, when possible, avoid extremes of temperature.

7 Do not jog if you have a cold, influenza, any form of stomach complaint or viral condition.

8 Wear proper footwear and clothing.

Suitable physical activities for the development of cardiovascular fitness include walking, swimming and cycling as well as jogging.

4 The cool-down a Perform exercises in a relaxed, non-stressed way.

b Spend no more than 5–10 minutes on this phase, depending on your fitness level.

c The heart rate should show adequate recovery by the end of the cool-down.

Suitable exercises for the cool-down phase include:

1 Gentle jogging and walking

2 Trunk side bends

3 Many relaxing flexibility exercises

4 Deep breathing with hands on hips

Further opportunities for your exercise programme

During the past decade there has been a tremendous growth of fitness clubs, health spas, weight control centres and other similar businesses to meet the increasing demand from the public.

Many people who are interested in trying to improve their health related fitness can develop their own programmes. The principles and guidelines in this book demonstrate how. There is no need to join a fitness club. However, some people may benefit enormously from them. If you enjoy the comfort of a well-equipped centre, the sociability and support of other people while exercising or dieting, or the guidance of a qualified exercise specialist, then these organizations may suit you. But bear in mind that some clubs are more professionally run than others. The following points are worth considering before joining:

1 You are making a long-term commitment when you join. You must use the facilities on a regular basis to gain the rewards you require.

2 To ensure regularity of training, and to save on travelling expenses, be sure that the centre is located conveniently.

3 Visit the centre before joining. Check the equipment and facilities. Do they suit your requirements? Is there an opportunity for a trial basis such as two weeks at a reduced rate?

4 Seek information about the qualifications of personnel and the individual exercise specialists. Are there any links with the medical profession?

5 Check the availability of use. For example, if you work on shifts, you might want to know about flexible working arrangements. Visit peak hour operations of the facility. Is it too overcrowded for your programme?

6 What are the membership fees? Are there any additional costs to use facilities such as the multi-gym?

7 Be careful of organisations that guarantee extremely rapid physical fitness gains or weight loss programmes. As you know, this needs to be achieved over a period of time.

If you think about these points, it should enable you to determine whether or not a particular centre or club meets your requirements. Organisations that are professionally run can be extremely helpful in guiding you through your health related fitness programme. Unprofessional centres may give you little in return for your hard-earned money.

In conclusion, the results of enjoyable hard work and determination, will more than repay your efforts. However, your efforts will be in vain if you stop when you reach your goal. You will lose all the health related fitness as fast as you gained it if you do not continue the programme. It is an ongoing lifetime commitment you are undertaking. Make this commitment now.

Bibliography

American Alliance for Health, Physical Recreation and Dance. *AAHPERD Health Related Fitness Test Manual*. AAHPERD publications, Washington DC, 1980.

Allsen, P. et al. *Fitness for Life: an individualized approach*. Wm. C. Brown Publishers, Dubuque, Iowa, 3rd edition, 1984.

Almond, L. 'Health Related Fitness in Schools'. *Bulletin of Physical Education*, Vol. 19, No. 2, 1983.

Astrand, P. O., and Rodahl, K. *Textbook of work physiology*. McGraw-Hill, New York, 2nd edition, 1977.

Baun, W. B., et al. 'A nomogram for the estimate of percent body fat from generalized equations'. *Research Quarterly for Exercise and Sport*, Vol. 52: pp. 380–384, 1981.

Beaulieu, J. E. *Stretching for All*. The Athletic Press, Pasadena, California, 1980.

Cooper, K. H. *The Aerobics Way*. M. Evans and Co., New York, 1977.

Corbin, C. and Lindsey, R. *Concepts of Physical Fitness with Laboratories*. Wm. C. Brown Publishers, Dubuque, Iowa, 5th edition, 1985.
Fitness for Life. Scott, Foresman and Co., Glenview, Illinois, 2nd edition, 1983.

Davis, A. *Looking After Yourself*. The Health Education Council, 1979.

De Vries, H. A. *Physiology of Exercise for Physical Education and Athletics*. Wm. C. Brown Publishers, New York, 3rd edition, 1980.

Fleishman, E. A. *The Structure and Measurement of Physical Fitness*. Prentice-Hall Inc., Englewood Cliffs, N.J., 1964.

Fodor, R. and Taylor, G. *Junior Body Building*. Sterling Publishing Co. Ltd., Poole, Dorset, 1979.

Getchell, B. *Physical Fitness – a way of life*. John Wiley and Sons, New York, 1983.

Jacobson, E. *You Must Relax*. McGraw-Hill, New York, 1976.

Karpovich, P. and Sinning, W. *Physiology of Muscular Activity*. W. B. Saunders Co., now Holt-Saunders, Eastbourne, E. Sussex, 1971.

Kraus, H. and Raab, W. *Hypokinetic Disease*. C. C. Thomas, Springfield, Illinois, 1961.

Madders, J. *Stress and Relaxation*. Martin Dunitz Ltd., London, 1980.

Sharkey, B. *Physiology and Physical Activity*. Harper and Row, New York, 1975.
Physiology of Fitness. Human Kinetics Publishers, Champaign, Illinois, 1979.

Tancred, W. and Tancred, G. *Weight Training for Sport.* Hodder and Stoughton Educational, Sevenoaks, Kent, 1984.

Watson, A. *Physical Fitness and Athletic Performance.* Longman Group Limited, Harlow, Essex, 1983.

Westcott, W. *Strength Fitness.* Allyn and Bacon, Inc., Boston, Mass., 1983.

Williams, M. *Lifetime Physical Fitness.* Wm. C. Brown Publishers, Dubuque, Iowa, 1985.

Index